Introduct

Simple Weekly Meal Plans – Volume 1 contains four weeks of menu plans on The Hallelujah Diet, which help maintain variety for you and your family *(Simple Weekly Meal Plans – Volume 2 contains an additional four weeks)*. With both books, you can literally go for eight weeks and never have the same meal twice!

These recipes contain relatively few ingredients, the instructions are easy to follow, and best of all, they taste great and are good for you, too! Most of the menus can be prepared in less than one hour. This is a big plus for busy people, whether you work at home or away from home.

If you are just starting The Hallelujah Diet and the thought of preparing several weeks worth of new menus overwhelms you, here is another simple idea that may work better for you:
- Go through the Simple Weekly Meal Plans books and mark some of the recipes you think your family would like.
- Plan seven different simple menus
- Prepare the same menu on a given day of the week; for instance, Monday nights could be brown rice and steamed vegetable night, Tuesday nights could be baked potato and salad night, Wednesday nights could be Layered Mexican Casserole night, etc. – you get the idea.

Of course, it is a given that each meal would begin with a large garden salad with green, leafy lettuce as the base for your salad. Especially for those homes where both husband and wife may be late getting home in the afternoon after a long, busy day, implementing this plan will make meal preparation less stressful for everybody. On the weekends and holidays, you could try out a new recipe or two for your family and of course, remember to put a star by the ones that are "keepers"!

NOTE: The recipes in this book generally feed three to four people; if your family is larger, you can easily double all of the recipes.

The nutritional and health information in this book is based on the teachings of God's Holy Word, the Bible, as well as research and personal experience by the author and others. The purpose of this book is to provide information and education about health. The author and publisher do not directly or indirectly dispense medical advice or prescribe the use of diet as a form of treatment for sickness without medical approval. Nutritionists and other experts in the field of health and nutrition hold widely varying views. The author and publisher do not intend to diagnose or prescribe. The author and publisher intend to offer health information to help you cooperate with your doctor or other health practitioners in your mutual quest for health. In the event you use this information without your doctor or other health practitioner's approval, you prescribe for yourself. This remains your constitutional right. The author and publisher assume no responsibility.

Authored by Marilyn Polk
Hallelujah Acres extends special thanks to Hallelujah Acres Health Minister Marilyn Polk for her tireless efforts in researching, testing and compiling the recipes in *Simple Weekly Meal Plans – Volume 1* and *Simple Weekly Meal Plans – Volume 2*.

In 1999, Marilyn discovered The Hallelujah Diet, which freed her from four long years of suffering with fibromyalgia. To this day, she remains symptom-free. It was this life-changing experience that led her and her husband Doug to pursue Health Minister training in 2000. Today, Marilyn and Doug Polk are still among the most progressive and influential Health Ministers in Hallelujah Acres history.

First printing 2005
Revised 2010

ISBN 978-0929619194

This edition published and distributed by

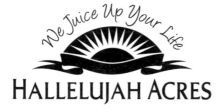

Hallelujah Acres Inc.
P.O. Box 2388 • Shelby, NC 28151
704-481-1700 • www.hacres.com

Week One

GROCERY LIST

First of all, rid your kitchen of unhealthy foods. Throw them away if they are already opened; take them to a food pantry or soup kitchen in your area if the products are unopened.

This list includes only the foods you will need for each recipe; in other words, no extra fruits or veggies are listed for snacking. Once a spice is listed on a grocery list, it will not be listed again since spices generally will last for several weeks. Always purchase organic spices since they have not been irradiated.

Purchase organic foods when available. Also, since everyone has different salad preferences, the term "your favorite salad ingredients" is the first item on the grocery list each week. Because The Hallelujah Diet includes a large amount of raw food, two or three trips to the grocery store each week is not uncommon.

The first week's grocery list will be the longest because you will be stocking your pantry with several items that you will not need to purchase each week. Note that breakfast foods for children are not included on the weekly lists.

RAW VEGETABLES:

lettuces*	broccoli florets *(2 packages)*	carrots
celery	2 onions	1 red onion
spinach *(2 packages)*	fresh basil *(1/2 cup)*	4 corn on the cob
2 red peppers	2 yellow peppers	parsley
scallions *(1 bunch)*	9 new red potatoes	garlic
4 yellow squash	6 zucchini	mushrooms
1 cauliflower	1 avocado	

NOTE: Shop for a variety of lettuces such as red leaf, green leaf, Romaine, Boston, baby, etc. (never use iceberg lettuce because it contains very little nutrition and does not digest well).

OPTIONAL VEGETABLES FOR WEEK ONE:

radishes	beets
sweet potato	cabbage

FRUITS:

apples	oranges	bananas
berries	grapes *(large bunch)*	peaches
raisins	watermelon	cantaloupe
honeydew melon	3 cucumbers	blueberries *(2 boxes)*
tomatoes	strawberries *(2 packages)*	

OPTIONAL FRUITS FOR WEEK ONE:

plums	grapefruit	pineapple
cherries	pears	mangoes

*NUTS AND SEEDS:

almonds	walnuts	pecans
macadamias	sunflower seeds	sesame seeds
pumpkin seeds	flaxseed	pine nuts

*NOTE: Buy raw nuts and soak them for about 8 hours in distilled water. Drain. Then put them on teflex sheets and dehydrate for about 6 hours at 104 degrees or lower. Soaking allows the enzymes to be released in the nuts and also washes away phytic acids, which interfere with calcium absorption. Nuts which have been soaked and dehydrated taste so much better than just eating them out of the package.

MISCELLANEOUS/STAPLES:

whole-wheat spaghetti	brown or basmati rice
multi-grain cornbread mix by Arrowhead Mills	bulgur wheat
Muir Glen diced tomatoes w/ basil and garlic (3)	pita pockets
tri-color pasta	wheat sub bread
100% stone ground whole-wheat bread	whole-wheat flour
unbleached bread flour	raw, unfiltered honey
Westbrae Natural dijon mustard	Vegenaise
dried red beans	grapeseed oil
flaxseed oil and/or olive oil	lentils
frozen chopped spinach (1 box)	salsa
Muir Glen diced tomatoes with green chilies (2)	Celtic Sea Salt
pineapple tidbits in its own juice	garlic powder
Simply Organic SW Taco Mix	agar-agar
curry powder	paprika
onion flakes	dill weed
Bragg's apple cider vinegar	water chestnuts
canned organic kidney beans	sage
canned organic black-eye peas	black olives (sliced)
canned organic black beans	baked tortilla chips
Earth Balance margarine substitute (optional)**	yeast
Ener-G Egg Replacement	oregano
frozen green peas (1 package)	herb seasoning
frozen corn niblets (1 package)	couscous

MISCELLANEOUS/STAPLES *(continued)*:

organic butter *(optional)*
Fantastic Foods Spinach Parmesan Hummus
organic tomato sauce
Vegan Rella cheese substitutes *(optional)***

organic apple juice
Rice Dream milk
currants
chives

**CHEESE AND BUTTER SUBSTITUTES

Because most Americans eat a lot of cheese and margarine or butter, this list includes some substitutes, but please realize that for optimum health, you really need to eliminate these foods from your diet as soon as possible. Most rice, almond, and soy cheese substitutes contain an animal derivative, casein.

For recipes calling for butter or margarine, you can substitute a butter blend. The recipe is as follows: 1 stick of organic butter, 4-8 tablespoons of olive or flaxseed oil, and 1 teaspoon of raw honey. Blend until smooth. Another option is to use Earth Balance, which can be found at your local health food store. Please use these products in moderation and have as your goal to eliminate them from your diet as soon as possible.

NOTES: _____

_____

_____

_____

_____

_____

_____

_____

_____

_____

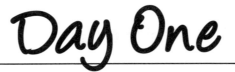

LUNCH:
Large Garden Salad

LARGE GARDEN SALAD
The Hallelujah Diet recommends a large vegetable salad for lunch at least three times per week. The base of any great salad is a variety of greens, such as red or green leaf lettuce, romaine lettuce, endive, spinach, etc. Add 5-6 vegetables, preferably organic, from the following list and top with your favorite homemade dressing. *(See Salad Dressing section for recipes.)*

Salad Ingredients

sliced cucumbers	diced yellow, red, or orange peppers
mushrooms	diced tomatoes or cherry tomatoes
chopped celery	raw, sweet corn
diced sweet onion	broccoli florets
cauliflower florets	sliced avocado
sliced radishes	grated carrots
grated beet	grated sweet potato
julienned zucchini	julienned yellow squash
organic raisins	fresh sprouts
grated red cabbage	frozen corn niblets *(rinsed in colander)*
diced apples	frozen green peas

Toppings

raw sesame seeds	raw sunflower seeds*
raw pumpkin seeds	chopped, raw walnuts
chopped, raw pecans	sliced, raw almonds
pine nuts	

*Grind seeds in a coffee grinder and sprinkle on top of salad.

DINNER:
Broccoli Salad #1, Judy's Red Beans and Rice, Cornbread

BROCCOLI SALAD #1

3/4 cup of Vegenaise*, or homemade almond mayonnaise**   4 cups broccoli florets
2 Tbsp fresh lemon juice   2 Tbsp raw honey
1/2 cup organic raisins   1/4 cup raw sunflower seeds

Mix mayonnaise substitute, honey, lemon juice, seeds, and raisins. Pour over florets and stir well.

NOTE: Grapeseed Oil Vegenaise is egg free, dairy free, cholesterol free, and preservative free, but it contains 90 calories per tablespoon.

DINNER *(continued)*:
Broccoli Salad #1, Judy's Red Beans and Rice, Cornbread

**Almond Mayonnaise

1/2 cup almonds, soaked overnight
2 tsp onion flakes
1 Tbsp agar-agar - *not necessary*
1 lemon, juiced

3/4 cup distilled water
1/4 tsp Celtic Sea Salt
3 pitted dates

Mix all of the above ingredients in your food processor. After well blended, slowly pour in 1/2 cup cold-pressed extra virgin olive oil while continuing to blend. *(This recipe can be used in all recipes calling for Vegenaise.)*
└ *try 1/4*

JUDY'S RED BEANS and RICE

3 or 4 cloves finely chopped garlic
2 or 3 jalapeno or other hot pepper *(optional)*
1 cup chopped celery
1 tsp Celtic Sea Salt
1 can organic chopped tomatoes *(optional)*

1 pound package red beans
1 cup chopped onion
1 cup chopped red pepper
1 cup uncooked brown rice

Soak red beans in distilled water over night. Drain and rinse thoroughly. Place beans in a large pot, cover with distilled water, and bring to a boil. Add remaining ingredients, except rice. Reduce heat to simmer. Cook two hours stirring occasionally or put in your crock-pot and allow to cook all day.

To prepare brown or basmati rice, boil 2 cups distilled water and 1 teaspoon of Celtic Sea Salt. Add 1-1/3 cups of rice, reduce heat, and simmer for 30 minutes without lifting the lid. Set off stove and let sit for 15 minutes. Fluff with fork and serve beans over rice.

CORNBREAD

2 cups Whole-Grain Cornbread Mix by Arrowhead Mills
1-1/4 cups distilled water or Rice Dream milk replacement
1 egg substitute*
2 Tbsp raw honey
2 Tbsp grapeseed oil

Stir all ingredients together. Pour into oiled (olive) eight-inch pan. Bake at 400 degrees for 30-40 minutes or until golden brown.

*Egg Substitute: Ener-G Replacement (Can be purchased at health food store)
—or— 1/4 cup ground flaxseed, 3/4 cup pure water

Add water to flaxseed. Blend on high for 2-3 minutes. Chill for 1 hour. 1 egg = 1/4 cup of the flaxseed mixture

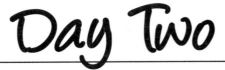

LUNCH:
Stuffed Pita Pocket

STUFFED PITA POCKET
Use Spinach Parmesan Hummus mix by Fantastic Foods *(non-GMO)*. It only takes a few of minutes to prepare. Stuff with such vegetables as diced tomatoes, lettuce, diced onion, sliced cucumbers, sprouts, grated carrot, red pepper strips, and salsa.

DINNER:
Spinach Salad with Simple Dressing, Skillet Italian Casserole

SPINACH SALAD WITH SIMPLE DRESSING
This recipe is from Kim Wilson's book, *Everyday Wholesome Eating...In the Raw*, available from Hallelujah Acres.

3 Tbsp olive oil
1 Tbsp honey
1 garlic clove, crushed
large bunch of spinach
1/3 cup pine nuts, walnuts, or chopped
    walnuts or chopped almonds *(optional)*
red onion

2 Tbsp apple cider vinegar
1/4 sweet onion, chopped
1/2 tsp sea salt
1 avocado, sliced
cherry tomatoes
oil-cured olives

Mix first six ingredients and allow to marinate at least for a few hours. Break up spinach and serve on plates topped with avocado, nuts, and optional toppings. Drizzle with dressing.

SKILLET ITALIAN CASSEROLE
2 cups tri-color pasta
1 cup chopped onion
2 cups frozen, chopped spinach, thawed
1 can organic tomatoes with garlic and basil
1/2 tsp garlic powder
1/3 cup organic Parmesan Veggie topping *(optional)*
1/2 cup shredded cheese substitute* *(optional)*

1 tsp Celtic Sea Salt
1 stalk celery, diced
3 carrots, sliced
1 can organic tomato sauce
1/2 tsp oregano
1/2 cup sliced mushrooms

Boil pasta in salted water. Meanwhile, steam sauté onion, celery, carrots, and mushrooms in 1/4 cup of water over medium heat for about 5 minutes. Add sauce, tomatoes, garlic powder, oregano, veggie topping, and drained pasta. Simmer for 10 additional minutes. Remove from heat and add spinach. Stir thoroughly and top with shredded "cheese."

Day Three

LUNCH:
Fruit Plate or Melon Plate

FRUIT PLATE OR MELON PLATE
Include such fruits as apple slices, orange sections, banana, red grapes, sliced kiwi, sliced peaches, strawberries, blueberries, raspberries, etc. Don't mix melons with any other fruit as they digest more quickly than other fruits. Mix melons such as watermelon, honeydew, cantaloupe, etc.

DINNER:
Spinach Salad #1, Savory Rice, Snappy Salsa

SPINACH SALAD #1
1 package organic baby spinach   6–7 Medjool dates*, chopped
1 diced apple   1/2 cup chopped walnuts

Salad Dressing
1/2 cup raw honey
1/4 cup Westbrae Natural Dijon mustard
2 Tbsp flaxseed or olive oil

Blend dressing well and pour over salad just before serving.

NOTE: These are big, luscious dates, unlike those small ones you'll buy in packages. Most grocery stores now carry them; they can also be found at your local health food store or an international market.

SAVORY RICE
To prepare brown or basmati rice: Boil 2 cups of pure water and 1 teaspoon of Celtic Sea Salt. Stir in 1-1/3 cups of rice. Cover and simmer for 30 minutes. Remove from heat and let sit for 15 minutes.

2 celery ribs, chopped   2 sliced green onions
1 can water chestnuts drained and chopped   1/4 tsp sage
1/3 cup sliced almonds   1/2 tsp parsley

While rice is cooking, sauté celery and onions in 2–3 tablespoons of water for about 3 minutes. Add the water chestnuts, sage, and parsley. Sauté for 2 minutes longer. Stir almonds into rice and serve.

DINNER *(continued)*:
Spinach Salad #1, Savory Rice, Snappy Salsa

SNAPPY SALSA

2 cups corn niblets, fresh or frozen

1 carrot, shredded

1 can organic chopped tomatoes, drained

1/4 tsp paprika

1/2 tsp garlic powder

1 can organic black beans, drained*

1/3 cup diced, sweet onion

2 Tbsp diced, sweet pepper

1 tsp parsley

Put all of the above ingredients in a large bowl, add the dressing, and stir well.

Dressing

3 Tbsp lemon juice

2 Tbsp raw honey

1-1/2 Tbsp Westbrae Natural Dijon mustard

Serve with baked tortilla chips. If you double the dressing, this dish can also be served over brown rice.

NOTE: Because this cookbook is written especially for busy people, recipes include canned tomatoes and beans. Look for the organic variety with lined cans. Of course, a healthier alternative to canned beans would be to prepare the dried ones according to package directions. You would use 2 cups of cooked beans in this recipe.

Notes: _____

_____

_____

_____

_____

_____

_____

_____

_____

_____

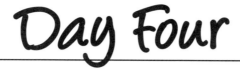

LUNCH:
Veggie Sub or Sandwich

VEGGIE SUB OR SANDWICH

Use wheat sub rolls or 100% stone ground whole-wheat bread. Spread a little grapeseed oil Vegenaise, or homemade almond mayonnaise *(see recipe)* on bread. Top with the vegetables of your choice.

Top with veggies like red leaf lettuce, baby spinach, sliced tomatoes, red bell pepper strips, shredded carrots, sliced cucumbers, fresh sprouts, shredded zucchini, black olives, and salsa.

NOTE: If you eat bread for lunch (never more than 1 whole sub roll or 2 sandwich slices), then don't eat any bread for dinner. Bread is a simple carbohydrate that turns to sugar very quickly in your system.

DINNER:
Garden Salad *(See Week One, Day One)*
Sula's Mixed Marinated Vegetables and Couscous, Super Squash

SULA'S MIXED MARINATED VEGETABLES and COUSCOUS

2 cups broccoli florets	1 cup chopped cauliflower
1 yellow squash, quartered and sliced	2 celery ribs, chopped
5 green onions, chopped or red onion rings	1/2 red bell pepper, julienned
kernels from 1 ear of sweet corn (raw)	1/4 cup chopped pecans or walnuts
1/4 cup parsley, chopped (can use dried)	1/2 tsp Celtic Sea Salt

Sula's Dressing

4 Tbsp flaxseed oil	3 Tbsp raw honey
1/2 tsp garlic powder	1/2 tsp onion flakes
1/4 cup lemon juice or Bragg's apple cider vinegar	

Pour the dressing over vegetables, mix well, and marinate at least one hour. Serve over couscous, which has been prepared according to package directions. This may be served alone as a raw salad.

SUPER SQUASH

5 medium zucchini, sliced or julienned	1 onion, sliced
3 medium yellow squash, sliced or julienned*	2 Tbsp distilled water
1 small red or orange pepper, julienned	1 tsp Celtic Sea Salt
1 minced garlic clove or 1 tsp minced garlic	dash of paprika

Sauté vegetables in covered skillet for about 12 minutes. Better yet, serve it raw!

*NOTE: A mandolin slicer, which can be purchased at a kitchen specialty store, is ideal to julienne your vegetables.

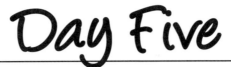

LUNCH:
Blended Salad

BLENDED SALAD

A blended salad enabled you to eat a larger volume of raw foods in less time, masticated much more efficiently, delivering much more nutritional value to the body with less energy expended on digesting.

1 tomato	1/4 cucumber (peel if not organic)
2 cups greens	1/4 bell pepper (not green)
1 stalk celery	1/2 avocado
1/2 cup broccoli florets	1/2 tsp herb seasoning

Place all ingredients in a blender and blend well.

DINNER:
Garden Salad *(See Day One)*, Vegetarian Pizza

VEGETARIAN PIZZA
1-1/2 cups distilled water
1-1/2 Tbsp grapeseed oil
1-1/2 Tbsp raw honey

Pour the above ingredients in your bread machine.

Add the following:
3-1/4 cups whole wheat flour
1/2 cups unbleached bread flour
1-1/2 tsp Celtic Sea Salt

Scoop a small hole on top of dry ingredients and pour 1-1/2 teaspoon of yeast in the hole. Set the machine to the "basic dough" setting and "start." After 1 hour 50 minutes, dump the dough onto a lightly floured pastry sheet. Divide into 2 balls and pat onto 2 pizza pans that have been lightly sprayed with olive oil. Let the dough sit for 15 minutes. Bake at 350 degrees for about 15 minutes or until golden brown.

Pizza Topping
Remove crust from oven and top with an organic pasta sauce. Add your favorite vegetables such as diced sweet onion, red and yellow pepper strips, mushrooms, broccoli florets, spinach, sliced zucchini, black olives, and thinly sliced tomatoes. Sprinkle shredded Mozzarella cheese substitute on top (optional) and heat for a couple of minutes in a warm oven until the cheese melts.

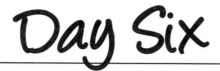

LUNCH:
Terrific Taco Salad

TERRIFIC TACO SALAD
1-1/2 cup distilled water
1/2 cup of Arrowhead Mills organic bulgur wheat
1/2 package Simply Organic Southwest Taco Mix

Bring water to a boil. Add bulgur wheat and taco mix. Stir, reduce heat to low, and simmer for 10 minutes. Remove from heat and let sit for 15 additional minutes.

Meanwhile in a large bowl mix the following:
1 head red or green lettuce, torn	1-2 carrots shredded
1 diced cucumber	2 tomatoes, diced
1/2 cup chopped onion	1/2 tsp garlic powder
1 can kidney beans, drained and rinsed	1/2 cup salsa
2 handfuls baked tortilla chips, crushed	2/3 cup shredded "cheese" *(optional)*

Add bulgur wheat mixture to the vegetables.

Mix well and top with 2/3 cup shredded "cheese."

DINNER:
Broccoli Salad #2, Spicy Lentils, Creamy New Potatoes

BROCCOLI SALAD #2
4 cups broccoli florets	1 cup red grapes, halved
1/3 cup chopped red onion	2 ribs celery, chopped

Dressing
3/4 cup Vegenaise, or almond mayonnaise *(See Day One, Dinner)*
1 Tbsp Bragg's apple cider vinegar
2 Tbsp raw honey

Mix dressing and pour over salad. Stir well.

SPICY LENTILS
1 cup lentils	1-1/2 cups distilled water
1 small onion, chopped	2 cloves of garlic, minced
1 can organic diced tomatoes w/ green chilies	1 tsp Celtic Sea Salt

Put lentils, water, onion, garlic, and salt in pot and cook on medium heat for 30 minutes. Add tomatoes. Reduce heat and simmer for 10 additional minutes.

CREAMY NEW POTATOES

8–9 new red potatoes, scrubbed
3 Tbsp Earth Balance margarine substitute*
2 Tbsp Vegenaise or almond mayo
1 tsp lemon juice

1 tsp Celtic Sea Salt
1/2 tsp dill weed
1 Tbsp chives

Put potatoes and salt in pot with distilled water. Bring to a boil, and then simmer until tender. Drain. Add butter. Combine remaining ingredients and add to potatoes, mixing well.

Notes: _____

_____

_____

_____

_____

_____

_____

_____

_____

_____

_____

_____

_____

_____

_____

_____

_____

Day Seven

LUNCH:
Large Garden Salad *(See Week One, Day One)*
Meatless Spaghetti

MEATLESS SPAGHETTI
This meal is super easy! Fill a pot with water and 1 teaspoon of Celtic Sea Salt. Bring to a boil and then add whole-wheat spaghetti or angel hair. Put a lid on pot, reduce heat, and simmer for 10-12 minutes, or until pasta is tender. Drain. Top with Parmesan flavor Veggie Topping by Galaxy Foods *(optional)*. Serve with wholegrain bread.

IMPORTANT: Because pasta is not a low calorie food, keep the serving small.

DINNER:
Large Garden Salad *(See Week One, Day One)*
Orzo and Wild Rice

ORZO and WILD RICE
16 oz pkg orzo	8 oz pkg Lundberg Organic Quick Wild Rice
1 yellow pepper, diced	1/2 cup almonds, cut lengthwise*
1 red pepper, diced	3 ears of fresh corn niblets
1/2 cup red onion, diced	1/2 cup scallions, sliced thin *(green part only)*
1/2 cup currants	

Cook orzo *(found in the pasta section of your grocery store)* and rice by directions on package. For an all-raw dish, the orzo and rice could be soaked for 1-1/2 days. Blend all ingredients with basil vinaigrette well in a large bowl. Cover and refrigerate until ready to serve.

BASIL VINAIGRETTE
1/2 cup basil leaves (loosely-packed)*	2 garlic cloves
1/4 cup white balsamic vinegar	1/4 tsp sea salt
or Bragg's apple cider vinegar	1/4 cup olive oil *(or flaxseed oil)*
1 tsp dry mustard	
or Westbrae Natural Dijon mustard	

Put everything except oil in blender and pulse until just blended. Slowly add oil till blended. Pour over orzo and wild rice.

NOTE: You can buy a potted basil plant and set it on your patio for full sun. These plants are so easy to grow. Pick large leaves, rinse, pat dry, and dehydrate. Store in a freezer bag in a dark place and enjoy basil all winter long.

NOTES:

Week Two

GROCERY LIST

carrots
1 red pepper
green onions
baking potatoes
3 zucchini
mushrooms
2 lemons
dates
raisins
kelp
basil
flaxseed oil
dough enhancer
dried black beans
whole grain buns
pita pockets
Spectrum Naturals
    Zesty Italian dressing

1 red onion
celery
6 red potatoes
salad greens
3 yellow squash
1 cauliflower
1 lime
olives
3 cucumbers
parsley
chives
frozen corn niblets
tri-color pasta (2 pkgs)
instant brown rice
Angostura Worcestershire
liquid lecithin
unbleached bread flour

1 yellow pepper
broccoli florets
baby spinach
cabbage (2 heads)
sweet potatoes
red grapes
apples
tomatoes
cherry tomatoes
dill weed
walnuts
fresh corn
frozen green peas
whole-grain bread
old-fashioned oats
wheat berries
wheat gluten

Notes: _____

_____

_____

_____

_____

_____

_____

_____

_____

_____

_____

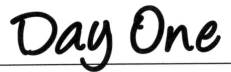

Day One

LUNCH:
Better Than Tuna

BETTER THAN TUNA *(adapted from Rhonda Malkmus' book, Recipes for Life from God's Garden)*

1 small bag of organic carrots
1/4 medium sweet onion

1/2 red bell pepper
2 stalks of celery

Process the above ingredients in a food processor until finely chopped. Pour in a bowl. Coarse-chop 1 tomato, strain, then add to bowl.

Blend in the following:
1/2 tsp Celtic Sea Salt
3 Tbsp Vegenaise or almond
  mayonnaise *(See Day One, Dinner)*

1 Tbsp parsley
1/2 tsp kelp

Can be served in a whole-wheat pita pocket or on a bed of lettuce.

DINNER:
No Mayo Coleslaw, Fresh Sliced Tomatoes *(peel if not organic)*,
Warm Mustard Potato Salad, Corn on the Cob
(follow package directions)

NO MAYO COLESLAW
1 head of cabbage, shredded
1 cup of lettuce, thinly-sliced

1 large carrot, shredded
1/4 cup chopped onion

Dressing
3 Tbsp fresh lemon juice
3 Tbsp olive oil

3 Tbsp raw honey
1/2 tsp Celtic Sea Salt

WARM MUSTARD POTATO SALAD
5-6 red potatoes, peeled and diced
1/4 cup Westbrae Natural Dijon mustard
2 green onions, sliced
1 Tbsp dill weed
1/4 tsp fresh lime juice

3 Tbsp Vegenaise
1/2 cup chopped red onion
2 cloves garlic, minced
1/2 tsp Celtic Sea Salt

Cook potatoes in salt until tender. Meanwhile, mix other ingredients. Drain potatoes and add to dressing. Stir until well blended. Sprinkle with paprika.

Day Two

LUNCH:
Spinach Salad #2, Creamy Corn Salad

SPINACH SALAD #2

5 cups baby spinach
1 apple, diced
2 Tbsp sesame seeds
1 Tbsp grated orange peel

1/2 cup slivered almonds
1/2 cup organic raisins
1 green onion, chopped

Honey Mustard Dressing

1/4 cup Westbrae Natural Dijon mustard
2 Tbsp flaxseed oil or olive oil
1/3 cup raw honey

Mix dressing well and pour over salad just before serving.

CREAMY CORN SALAD

2 cups corn *(frozen niblets or fresh
  raw corn cut from the cob)*
1/3 cup Vegenaise

1 tomato, diced
1/2 cup chopped onion
1/4 tsp dill weed

DINNER:
Blended Salad *(See Week One, Day Five)*, Baked Potatoes

BAKED POTATOES

Cook whole potatoes *(one per person)* covered in water at low heat for 30 minutes. This cuts down on the high heat at which potatoes are normally baked. Bake one per person at 350 degrees until done. Top with lightly-steamed vegetables, flaxseed oil or Earth Balance, salsa, chives, and/or mushrooms.

Notes: _____

_____

_____

_____

_____

_____

_____

LUNCH:
Layered Basil Salad

LAYERED BASIL SALAD
Layer the following in a large glass bowl:

4 cups of assorted salad greens
2 cups cooked tri-color pasta
2 cups frozen green peas, rinsed in colander
1 cup broccoli florets

1 cup shredded carrots
1 cup diced red onion
2 cups chopped tomatoes

Dressing
1 cup Vegenaise
2 tsp Westbrae Natural Dijon mustard

1/2 tsp Celtic Sea Salt
1-1/2 tsp basil

Mix and spoon on top of salad. Show your kids/grandkids how to make a veggie "face" with black olives (eyes), sprouts (eyebrows), yellow pepper strip (nose), red pepper strip (mouth), spinach leaves (ears), or use whatever veggies you have on hand to make your own creation. It encourages reluctant children to eat the salad, too!

DINNER:
Coleslaw #1, Open-face Black Bean Burgers

COLESLAW #1
1 head of cabbage, shredded
1 large carrot, shredded
1 tsp parsley
1 Tbsp Vegenaise

1 apple, peeled and shredded
1/2 cup raisins*
1/2 tsp Celtic Sea Salt

Process the cabbage, apple, and carrot in your food processor using the S-blade. Combine all of the ingredients and mix well.

NOTE: Always use organic raisins as commercial raisins have been sprayed with pesticides and laid out in the sun to dry.

OPEN-FACE BLACK BEAN BURGERS
1 cup organic canned black beans
instant brown rice *(one serving)*
1/4 red pepper
1 carrot
1/2 Tbsp of freshly-ground flaxseed

1/4 tsp Celtic Sea Salt
1/2 onion
1 stalk of celery
1 slice of frozen whole grain bread
1 Tbsp of Angostura Worcestershire Sauce

Mash beans with a fork, leaving a few of them whole. Prepare instant brown rice for 1 person according to package directions. Use 1/2 cup of the cooked rice for your patties. Finely chop onion, red pepper, and celery. Grate carrot and frozen bread. Combine all of the above ingredients, add flaxseed and Worcestershire sauce and mix well.

Day Three

Form 8 patties and place on a cookie sheet that has been sprayed with olive oil. Bake for 10 minutes in a 350 degree oven. Remove, turn patties over, and bake 10 more minutes.

Put on a bed of lettuce *(or whole grain buns)* **and add your fixings:**
organic ketchup
tomato slices
fresh sprouts

Notes: _____

_____

_____

_____

_____

_____

_____

_____

_____

_____

_____

_____

_____

_____

_____

Day Four

LUNCH:
Colorful Veggie Salad

COLORFUL VEGGIE SALAD
2 carrots, chopped
1 cup corn, fresh or frozen
1/2 cup halved grape tomatoes

1 cup diced cucumber *(peel if not organic)*
1/4 cup chopped sweet onion
1/2 cup chopped red pepper

Dressing
2 Tbsp flaxseed oil
2 tsp raw honey
2 Tbsp fresh lemon juice

1 tsp onion flakes
1 tsp Italian herb seasoning

Mix vegetables and spoon on a bed of green leafy vegetables. Top with dressing.

DINNER:
Julienned Salad, Baked Sweet Potatoes

JULIENNED SALAD
2 zucchini, julienned *(use a mandolin)*
1/2 red pepper, julienned

2 yellow squash, julienned
1/3 cup sweet onion, cut in rings

Dressing
3 Tbsp flaxseed oil
1 tsp raw honey juice
1/2 tsp Celtic Sea Salt
1/2 tsp garlic powder

2 Tbsp apple cider vinegar or lemon
1/2 tsp dill weed
1 Tbsp Vegenaise

Combine vegetables. Mix dressing and pour over salad. Allow to marinate while potatoes are baking.

BAKED SWEET POTATOES
Cook whole potatoes covered in water at low heat for 30 minutes. This cuts down on the high heat at which potatoes are normally baked. Bake one per person at 350 degrees until done.

Possible toppings:
Flaxseed oil or Udo's Perfected Oil Blend
pure maple syrup
Earth Balance butter substitute
Cinnamon
Celtic Sea Salt and/or all-purpose seasoning (health food store)

Day Five

LUNCH:
Cauliflower Salad, Apple Slices

CAULIFLOWER SALAD
2-1/2 cups cauliflower, finely chopped
1/4 cup red pepper, diced
1 green onion, chopped
1/2 cup Spectrum Naturals
   Zesty Italian dressing
1 cup organic baby carrots, sliced
1 cup grape tomatoes, halved
1/3 cup organic raisins
1/3 cup walnuts, broken

Mix salad well and marinate for at least one hour before serving.

DINNER:
Garden Salad *(See Week One, Day One)*, Vegetarian Pizza

VEGETARIAN PIZZA *(same as Week One, Day Five – it's worth repeating!)*
1-1/2 cups distilled water
1-1/2 Tbsp grapeseed oil
1-1/2 Tbsp raw honey
Pour the above ingredients in your bread machine.

Add the following:
3-1/4 cups whole wheat flour
1/2 cups unbleached bread flour
1-1/2 tsp Celtic Sea Salt

Scoop a small hole on top of dry ingredients and pour 1-1/2 teaspoon of yeast in the hole. Set the machine to the "basic dough" setting and "start." After 1 hour 50 minutes, dump the dough onto a lightly floured pastry sheet. Divide into 2 balls and pat onto 2 pizza pans that have been lightly sprayed with olive oil. Let the dough sit for 15 minutes. Bake at 350 degrees for about 15 minutes or until golden brown.

Pizza Topping
Remove crust from oven and top with an organic pasta sauce. Add your favorite vegetables such as diced sweet onion, red and yellow pepper strips, mushrooms, broccoli florets, spinach, sliced zucchini, black olives, and thinly sliced tomatoes. Sprinkle shredded Mozzarella cheese substitute on top *(optional)* and heat for a couple of minutes in a warm oven until the cheese melts.

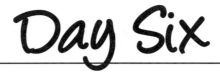

LUNCH:
Fruit Plate

FRUIT PLATE
Include such fruits as apple slices, orange sections, banana, red grapes, sliced kiwi, sliced peaches, strawberries, blueberries, raspberries, etc. Don't mix melons with any other fruit as they digest more quickly than other fruits.

DINNER:
Garden Salad *(use vegetables in this that are not in the lasagna)*, Very Veggie Lasagna, Nancy's Best Wheat Bread

VERY VEGGIE LASAGNA
Use uncooked rice or uncooked whole-wheat lasagna noodles. Spray 13 x 9 inch dish with olive oil. Pour a can of organic diced tomatoes with basil and garlic on bottom of dish. Place noodles next, then the following vegetables:

1 medium zucchini, sliced	2 yellow squash, sliced
1 small onion, diced	2 cups broccoli florets

Pour organic pasta sauce over above vegetables. You will need 1-1/2 - 2 jars of sauce for this recipe. Then put another layer of noodles over sauce. Put the following vegetables on next:

1 cup baby spinach	1 stalk celery, diced
1 cup pepper, diced *(red, orange, or yellow)*	1 cup mushrooms

Mix 1 clove of minced garlic and 1 teaspoon of Celtic Sea Salt with the remaining sauce. Pour over vegetables. Bake for 45 minutes, covered at 350 degrees. Remove from oven and shred some mozzarella cheese substitute and/or shake a little Parmesan Veggie Topping *(optional)* over all of this, too. Let stand 10 minutes before cutting. Serve with Nancy's Best Wheat Bread.

BEST WHEAT BREAD

1-1/2 cups pure water	2 Tbsp olive oil
1/3 cup raw honey	1 Tbsp liquid lecithin

Pour all of the above ingredients into your bread machine, then add the following dry ingredients:

1/2 cup unbleached bread flour	3-1/2 cups whole wheat flour
1 Tbsp wheat gluten	1/3 cup old fashioned oats
1-1/2 tsp Celtic Sea Salt	1 Tbsp freshly ground flaxseed
1 Tbsp dough enhancer *(optional)*	

Day Six

After adding the dry ingredients, scoop a small hole on top and add 2-1/2 teaspoons of yeast in the hole. Put the lid down and set for "basic" setting. Set crust on "light." Bread will be done in 3-1/2 hours. If you prefer 2 loaves, then set the machine for the "basic dough" setting. Remove after 1 hour 50 minutes.

Flour hands, dump dough onto floured surface, and cut in half. Form into balls and pat in 2 small loaf pans that have been sprayed with olive oil. Let rise in the oven at 120 degrees for 20 minutes only. Bake at 350 degrees until golden brown.

Notes: _____

_____

_____

_____

_____

_____

_____

_____

_____

_____

_____

_____

_____

_____

_____

_____

_____

Day Seven

LUNCH:
Rainbow Pasta Salad

RAINBOW PASTA SALAD
1 package tricolor pasta
1 cup chopped carrots
1 small cucumber, chopped
1 cup corn niblets, fresh or frozen

2 cups broccoli florets
1 tomato, chopped
1/4 cup chopped onion
1/2 tsp Celtic Sea Salt

Cook pasta according to package directions. Drain and rinse with cool water. Add vegetables and mix thoroughly. Pour 1 cup of Spectrum Naturals Zesty Italian dressing on salad. Stir and serve.

DINNER:
Veggie Subs

VEGGIE SUBS
Use whole wheat sub bread and provide a colorful array of vegetables to make the sandwiches.

Top with veggies such as:
sliced tomatoes
baby spinach
fresh sprouts
shredded carrots
black olives
diced onions

a variety of green, leafy vegetables
pepper strips
sliced cucumbers
shredded yellow squash
mushrooms
a variety of dressings

Notes: _____

_____

_____

_____

_____

_____

_____

Week Three

GROCERY LIST

red leaf lettuce cabbage *(1 head)*
6 beets
frozen mixed vegetables
1 avocado
green beans
oranges
pineapple chunks
strawberries *(2 packages)*
2 kiwi greens for salads
broccoli florets *(2 packages)*
bottled tomato juice
tomato sauce with chilies
Vegenaise
frozen green peas
maple syrup
whole wheat bread
apples
parsley
dry mustard
1 lime

carrots *(3 packages)*
4 lemons
raw almond butter*
frozen corn niblets
slivered almonds
cinnamon stick
bananas
red potatoes
sweet potatoes
4 zucchini
dried kidney beans
chili powder
basmati rice
avocado
broccoli
8 yellow squash
1 cucumber
scallions *(1 bunch)*
1 yellow pepper
spinach *(2 packages)*

2 onions
3 ears fresh corn
celery
almond cheese
dried basil
red grapes
tomatoes
white potatoes
barbecue sauce
1 red pepper
mushrooms
salsa
green onions
poppy seeds
coleslaw
grape tomatoes
quinoa
allspice
1 orange pepper

NOTE: This is a very pricey item if you purchase it at the health food store. You can make your own by soaking almonds with distilled water overnight. Drain, then feed the almonds through your Champion or Green Star Juicer with the blank plate on. You can add a little Udo's Oil or olive oil, Celtic Sea Salt, and/or raw honey.

Notes: _____

_____

_____

_____

_____

_____

_____

Day One

LUNCH:
Coleslaw #2, Rainbow Corn Salad, "Ants on a Log"

COLESLAW #2
2 cups leafy lettuce   2 carrots
head of cabbage   1/2 small onion

Put the above in your food processor and shred.

Dressing
1 tsp raw honey   1/2 tsp garlic powder
2/3 cup Vegenaise   1 tsp mustard
1/2 tsp Celtic sea salt

Mix well and blend into slaw. Sprinkle paprika on top.

RAINBOW CORN SALAD
2 cups corn niblets   1 cup diced red pepper
1 cup diced orange pepper   1 cup diced celery
1/2 cup green onions, chopped   1/4 cup parsley, minced
1/4 cup Parmesan Veggie topping *(optional)* 1 tsp cumin
1/2 tsp Celtic Sea Salt   dash of cayenne pepper

Dressing
2 Tbsp olive oil
3 Tbsp lime juice
2 garlic cloves, minced

"ANTS ON A LOG"
raw almond butter *(store bought or*   celery
   homemade – see Week Three grocery list) fruit spread *(optional)*
raisins

Slice celery into 2-inch strips. Fill with raw almond butter *(can blend in 100% fruit spread)* and top with raisins.

DINNER:
Garden Salad *(See Week One, Day One)*, Baked Squash
Green Bean Almandine

BAKED SQUASH
Choose a winter squash to bake. The directions for baking are on a label on the squash. Or if you choose the summer, yellow squash, then slice 6 squash, 1/3 cup chopped onion, 1/3 cup pure water, 1 tablespoon of grapeseed oil, and 1/2 teaspoon of Celtic sea salt. Cook on medium heat in a covered pot or skillet until tender.

GREEN BEAN ALMANDINE

3 cups green beans
1 tsp sea salt
1 tsp crushed basil
enough water to cover beans juice

2 tsp olive oil
1/4 tsp garlic powder
1 Tbsp fresh lemon

Cook the above ingredients on low heat with the lid on until beans are tender. During the last 5 minutes of cooking, add 3 tablespoons of slivered almonds.

Notes: _____

_____

_____

_____

_____

_____

_____

_____

_____

_____

_____

_____

_____

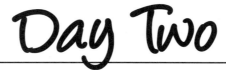

LUNCH:
Luscious Fruit Salad

LUSCIOUS FRUIT SALAD
1/2 cup fresh orange juice

1/4 cup raw honey

a little lemon zest

1/4 cup fresh lemon juice

a little orange zest

Bring the above ingredients to a boil, and then simmer for 5 minutes. Remove from heat.

Meanwhile cut up the following in a large bowl:
2 cups pineapple chunks

2 bananas, sliced

2 cups strawberries, sliced

1 cup red grapes (seeds removed)

2 oranges, sectioned and halved

2 kiwis, sliced

Pour cooled dressing over fruit and mix well.

DINNER:
Garden Salad *(See Week One, Day One)*, Nancy's Roasted Vegetables

NANCY'S ROASTED VEGETABLES
carrots

beets

sweet potatoes

potatoes

onions

rutabagas

Spray a large pan with olive oil. Cut up your favorite root vegetables, rub a little olive oil over vegetables and sprinkle lightly with Celtic Sea Salt. Only prepare one type of vegetable at a time and put in sections in your pan. Top the sweet potatoes with a dash of cinnamon. Roast, uncovered, at 375 degrees until tender (about 50 minutes).

Notes: _____

_____

_____

_____

_____

_____

LUNCH:
Scrumptious Pita Pockets

SCRUMPTIOUS PITA POCKETS
1 onion, chopped
2 medium zucchini, shredded
2 carrots, grated
3 Tbsp barbecue sauce*

1/2 red pepper, chopped
2 cups broccoli florets, chopped fine
2 Tbsp Vegenaise

Sauté onion and pepper in 3 tablespoons of pure water for about 3 minutes. Remove from heat and add remaining ingredients. Stuff pita bread 1/2 full with organic baby spinach and top with vegetable mixture.

Barbecue Sauce
(If you are in a hurry, just use store-bought sauce, but please read the label!)
This recipe is from the Hallelujah Food Show DVD "Holidays and Special Occasions."

1 cup tomatoes
1/4 cup chopped onion
1 tsp jalapeno
1 garlic clove
1 Tbsp olive oil

1/2 cup pitted organic Medjool dates
1/2 cup sun-dried tomatoes *(soaked, drained)*
1 tsp basil
1/2 tsp Celtic Sea Salt

Blend all of the above ingredients in your blender. *(I love my VitaMix for this.)*

DINNER:
Garden Salad *(See Week One, Day One)*, Chunky Chili

CHUNKY CHILI
4 cups tomato juice
1 onion, cut in rings
1 large potato, diced
1 zucchini, chopped
1/2 cup chopped red pepper
1 tsp Celtic Sea Salt
1 can organic tomato sauce with chilies

1/2 cup bulgur wheat
1/2 cup chopped carrots
1 jar mushrooms or 1/2 cup fresh & sliced
1-1/2 Tbsp chili powder
1-1/2 tsp cumin
1-1/2 cups cooked kidney beans*

Place all ingredients in a large pot. Bring to a boil and simmer for 1 hour, or put in your crock pot in the morning and cook all day.

NOTE: You can use organic kidney beans that have been drained. Better yet, soak a cup of beans overnight. Drain the next morning, put them in a pot, and cover with distilled water and 1/2 teaspoon Celtic Sea Salt. Cover and simmer for 1-1/2 hours. Let sit until you are ready to add the other ingredients that afternoon or cook with other ingredients in a crock-pot all day.

LUNCH:
Quick and Tasty Slaw, Layered Green Pea Salad

QUICK AND TASTY SLAW
1/2 package broccoli coleslaw
1/2 cup chopped walnuts
1/2 tsp Celtic Sea Salt

1 apple, shredded
1 tsp poppy seeds

Dressing
1-1/2 Tbsp fresh lemon juice or Bragg's apple cider vinegar
1-1/2 Tbsp olive, grapeseed, or Udo's oil
1-1/2 Tbsp pure maple syrup

Blend dressing well and pour over salad. Mix and serve.

LAYERED GREEN PEA SALAD
3 cups of greens, torn
1 cup celery, diced
1/2 cup chopped walnuts

1 cup green onions, finely chopped
2 cups frozen peas, rinsed

Layer salad and then spoon dressing over it.

Dressing
3/4 cup Vegenaise
1/3 cup Veggie Parmesan topping (optional)

2 Tbsp distilled water
1 Tbsp raw honey

DINNER:
Layered Mexican Casserole

LAYERED MEXICAN CASSEROLE
Layer the following in a 9" x 13" dish that has been lightly sprayed with olive oil.

1. 2 cups warm, mashed beans*
2. 3 wheat tortilla shells, warmed and cut into bite size pieces
3. Arrowhead Mills Organic Bulgur wheat prepared as follows:
   - Boil 1-1/2 cups of water.
   - Add 1/4 cup bulgur wheat and 1/4 package Simply Organic Taco Mix.
   - Simmer for 10 minutes.
   - Remove from heat and let set for 15 minutes.
4. Lettuce that has been torn *(Never use iceberg lettuce as it has very little nutrition.)*
5. Chopped tomatoes
6. Chopped onions
7. Sliced black olives
8. Salsa
9. Grated cheese substitute *(optional)*

*NOTE: If you are in a hurry, use the canned, vegetarian refried beans or organic black beans, reserving a little of the water and mash. A better choice would be to use dried black or turtle beans. Soak overnight, drain, cover with distilled water and 1/4 teaspoon Celtic Sea Salt, and simmer 1-1/2 hours. Mash with a little of the water and use in recipe.

Notes: _____

_____

_____

_____

_____

_____

_____

_____

_____

_____

_____

_____

_____

_____

_____

_____

_____

_____

_____

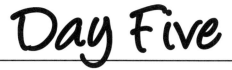

LUNCH:
Burritos Au Naturel

BURRITOS AU NATUREL
Using whole lettuce leaves, place as many of the following veggies as you desire. Top with salsa, fold up bottom and fold one side over the other.

shredded yellow squash
chopped tomatoes
chopped peppers
mushrooms

chopped onions
shredded zucchini
fresh alfalfa sprouts
avocado slices

DINNER:
Tabouli –OR– Cornbread Salad

TABOULI (from Everyday Wholesome Eating by Kim Wilson*)
2-3 cups cooked quinoa
2-3 diced tomatoes
1 bunch parsley, chopped
1/4 tsp allspice
2 scallions, sliced -OR- 1/4 sweet onion

1/3 cup olive oil
juice of 1 lemon
1/2 tsp sea salt
1/4 tsp cinnamon

optional ingredients:
1 cucumber, diced; 1/2 tsp dried mint

Mix oil, lemon juice, sea salt and cinnamon in a small bowl. Mix all other ingredients in larger bowl. Pour dressing from smaller bowl into large bowl and allow to marinate for an hour or more before serving.

This book can be ordered from Hallelujah Acres.

CORNBREAD SALAD
For cornbread recipe, see Day One, Dinner. Pour cornbread into 6 muffins tins lined with paper liners. Bake according to package directions.

Meanwhile mix the following in a large bowl:
2 large tomatoes, diced
4-6 cups of fresh greens
1/2 cup diced sweet onion
1 can of organic beans, rinsed
3 cornbread muffins, cooled*
3/4 cup organic salsa

1 cucumber diced (peel if not organic)
3 ears of fresh corn niblets
1 cup broccoli florets, cut small
1/4 cup sunflower seeds & drained
handful of fresh sprouts
2 carrots, shredded

Mix well. Use more muffins if you'd like or save some for another meal.

Day Six

LUNCH:
Carrot Salad, Spinach/Strawberry Salad

CARROT SALAD

2 cups shredded carrots
1/3 cup Vegenaise

1/2 cup organic raisins
1 shredded apple

SPINACH/STRAWBERRY SALAD

1 pound baby spinach
1/2 cup slivered almonds
2 Tbsp sesame seeds

2 cups sliced organic strawberries
2 Tbsp thinly-sliced green onions

Honey Mustard Dressing

1/4 cup Westbrae Natural Dijon mustard
2 Tbsp flaxseed oil or Udo's Oil
1/3 cup raw honey

Mix dressing well and pour on salad just before serving.

DINNER:
Basmati Rice Salad, Whole Grain Bread

BASMATI RICE SALAD
(Adapted from Recipes for Life from God's Garden by Rhonda Malkmus)
Bring 2 cups of distilled water and 1 teaspoon of Celtic Sea Salt to a boil. Stir in 1-1/3 cups of basmati rice. Cover and turn to lowest heat. Cook for 30 minutes without lifting the lid. Turn heat off and allow to sit for 15 additional minutes, covered.

While rice is cooking, prepare the following:

1 cup yellow squash, julienned
1 cup shredded carrots
1 cup broccoli florets
10 grape tomatoes, halved

1 cup zucchini, julienned
1/4 red pepper, chopped
1/2 cup green onions with tops

Dressing

1 lemon, juiced
2 Tbsp raw honey
1 Tbsp parsley

2 Tbsp olive oil
2 garlic cloves, minced
2 Tbsp dill

Pour dressing over vegetables and stir. Place spinach leaves around the perimeter of a platter. Spoon rice in the center and then pour vegetables in the middle of the rice. Cover and refrigerate for at least one hour. Serve with whole grain bread.

LUNCH:
You deserve a break today!

YOU DESERVE A BREAK TODAY!
Treat yourself and your family and go out to eat today. Choose a place that has a large salad and fruit bar. Load up on the fresh veggies. Look for a dressing that is low in calories and does not contain MSG; try some oil and a squeeze of lemon or just use a little salsa. Remember to avoid the mayonnaise salads.

DINNER:
Fresh Greens with Vinaigrette, Veggie Sandwich

FRESH GREENS WITH VINAIGRETTE
bowlful of fresh greens of your choice
1 cup diced red or yellow peppers
1/2 cup fresh basil, finely-chopped

1 cup sliced almonds
1/2 cup green onions
1/2 avocado, diced

Vinaigrette
1/4 cup Bragg's apple cider vinegar
1/4 tsp sea salt
1/4 cup flaxseed or olive oil

2 cloves garlic
1 tsp dry mustard

Put everything except oil in your blender. Blend and slowly add oil until well blended. Pour over salad just before serving.

VEGGIE SANDWICH
Enjoy a veggie sandwich on 100% stone ground whole wheat bread with your salad tonight. Load it with your favorite veggies.

Notes: _____

_____

_____

_____

_____

_____

_____

Week Four

GROCERY LIST

6+ apples
2 lemons
garlic
5 zucchini
tomatoes
baby carrots *(1 package)*
1 avocado
5 sweet potatoes
flaxseeds
minced onion
allspice
parsley
oregano
brown rice
vegetarian refried beans
tomatoes and chilies
veggie topping
frozen corn niblets
frozen vegetables for soup
pecans
organic ketchup
organic diced tomatoes

raisins
broccoli florets
4 onions
celery
grape tomatoes
lettuce spinach
2 yellow squash
7 red potatoes
sesame seeds
garlic powder
maple syrup
basil
rosemary
olive oil
olives
tomato juice
cheese substitute
organic butter
almond milk
walnuts
oranges
broccoli-cauliflower-carrot mix

dates
2 peppers
green onions
2 Portabella mushrooms
carrots *(3 packages)*
1 cucumber
1 cauliflower
sunflower seeds
agar-agar
cinnamon
vanilla
cayenne pepper
rolled oats
salsa
water chestnuts
pineapple tidbits *(1 can)*
Vegenaise
frozen green peas
persimmons
10 Roma tomatoes
2 zucchini

Notes: _____

_____

_____

_____

_____

_____

_____

_____

_____

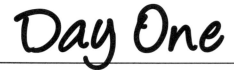

LUNCH:
Waldorf Salad, Garden Salad

WALDORF SALAD
This recipe was taken from the Hallelujah Acres Food Show video, Holidays and Special Occasions. The video can be ordered individually or as part of a set. Call 1-800-915-9355 to order.

2 apples, cubed	1/2 cup chopped celery
1/2 cup soaked walnuts	1/2 cup organic raisins
1 cup almond mayonnaise *(See Week One, Day One, Dinner)*	

Mix well and serve on a bed of lettuce.

DINNER:
Vegetable Soup*, Cornbread *(See Week One, Day One, Dinner)*

VEGETABLE SOUP

3/4 cup chopped onion	2 cloves minced garlic
1 rib chopped celery	1/2 cup frozen corn niblets
1/2 cup frozen green peas	1 tsp Celtic Sea Salt
1 can organic diced tomatoes	2 red potatoes, diced
large bottle tomato juice	1 small package frozen vegetables for soup
2/3 cup frozen lima beans	1 small jar sliced mushrooms

Simmer soup for 1-1/2 hours or put everything in your crock-pot in the morning and let it simmer all day.

Notes: _____

_____

_____

_____

_____

_____

_____

Day Two
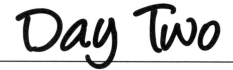

LUNCH:
Cruciferous Salad, Sliced Tomatoes

CRUCIFEROUS SALAD

2 cups cauliflower florets	2 cups broccoli florets
1 stalk chopped celery	1/2 cup chopped water chestnuts
2 chopped green onions	2/3 cup frozen peas, rinsed and drained

Dressing

1 cup Vegenaise	1 Tbsp raw honey
1/4 tsp Celtic Sea Salt	1 tsp fresh lemon juice
1 Tbsp Parmesan Veggie Topping *(optional)*	

Mix dressing well and blend into salad.

DINNER:
Garden Salad *(See Week One, Day One, Lunch)*
Honey-glazed Carrots, Parmesan Potatoes

HONEY-GLAZED CARROTS

2 cups baby carrots	2 Tbsp organic, unsalted butter
1/2 tsp Celtic Sea Salt	1 tsp fresh lemon juice
4 Tbsp raw honey	

Cook carrots in salted water on low heat until tender. When done, pour into a colander. In same pot, bring butter, honey, and juice to a boil. Reduce heat, add carrots, and simmer for 5-10 minutes, basting several times.

PARMESAN POTATOES

4-5 red potatoes, sliced in rounds	1 small onion, thinly sliced
2 Tbsp Earth Balance or butter blend	1/4 cup Parmesan Veggie
1/2 tsp Celtic Sea Salt Topping	1/2 tsp garlic powder

Spray a square baking dish with olive oil. Layer potatoes, onion rings, topping, salt, and powder. Dot margarine substitute on top, cover, and bake for 30-35 minutes at 350 degrees.

Notes: _____

_____

_____

Day Three

LUNCH:
Stuffed Tomatoes, Celery and Carrot Sticks

STUFFED TOMATOES

3 cups walnuts
1/4 sweet onion
1 Tbsp parsley
1 tsp Celtic Sea Salt

2 garlic cloves
1 stalk celery
1 Tbsp fresh lemon juice
1 Tbsp raw honey

Mix in your food processor using the S-blade. Put a large lettuce leaf on each plate. Take a large tomato, core the stem end, and cut into wedges, stopping 1/2 inch from the bottom. Stuff with nut spread and serve with celery and carrot sticks. This nut spread tastes great on pita bread, too.

DINNER:
Spinach Salad with Simple Dressing *(See Week One, Day Two, Dinner)*, Lemon Broccoli, Mashed Sweet Potatoes

LEMON BROCCOLI

1 bunch broccoli spears
2 cloves minced garlic
2 tsp grated organic lemon peel

1 small onion, chopped
1/2 tsp Celtic Sea Salt
1-1/2 tsp fresh lemon juice

Lightly steam broccoli for 3-5 minutes. Meanwhile sauté onion and garlic in 3 tablespoons of distilled water with lid on. Drain broccoli and add lemon peel, salt, onion, garlic, and juice.

MASHED SWEET POTATOES

Peel, cube, and cook 4 sweet potatoes on medium heat in distilled water until tender. Remove potatoes and save water. Put potatoes and 1/3 cup of the water in a large mixing bowl.

Add the following:

1/3 cup raw honey or pure maple syrup
3 Tbsp Earth Balance or butter blend
1 tsp Frontier vanilla
1/2 cup organic raisins

Blend potatoes, honey, Earth Balance, and vanilla well with your mixer. Add additional water if needed for the potatoes to be soft. Stir in raisins. Spoon into a square baking dish and sprinkle some chopped pecans on top.

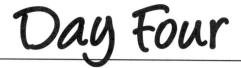

LUNCH:
Sunshine Salad, Delightful Green Salad

SUNSHINE SALAD

2 carrots, grated
2 yellow squash, grated
1 Tbsp pure maple syrup

1 sweet potato, grated
2 oranges, peeled and diced

Mix well and thank the good Lord for this life-giving salad.

DELIGHTFUL GREEN SALAD

greens of your choice
1 cup grape tomatoes sliced olives
1/4 cup sesame seeds ground in coffee grinder

1/2 cup chopped red peppers
1/3 cup pine nuts

Dressing

1 avocado
1/4 tsp Celtic Sea Salt
1 tsp basil

2 tomatoes, peeled
1/2 tsp oregano
2 cloves minced garlic

Blend ingredients well and pour over salad.

DINNER: Sun Burgers

SUN BURGERS

This recipe is taken from the Hallelujah Acres' Food Show Video, *Eating In The Outdoors*. These videos are loaded with lots of recipes.

Start dehydrating the patties around noon. Can be served between lettuce leaves or on whole-wheat buns.

1-1/4 cups carrots
4 Tbsp purified water
1/2 tsp Celtic Sea Salt

1-1/2 Tbsp ground flaxseeds
1 cup sunflower seeds
1 Tbsp

Process carrots using 'S' blade. Mix ground flaxseeds and 3 tablespoons of purified water. Grind sunflower seeds, sea salt, and 1 tablespoon purified water in your food processor.

Pour all of the above ingredients in a large bowl. Add the following and mix well:

1/3 cup chopped celery
2 Tbsp red pepper

1/3 cup chopped onion
2 Tbsp parsley

Form mixture into patties *(approximately 1/4 cup per patty)* and place on a Teflex sheet. Dehydrate for 4 hours on 106 degrees. Remove from dehydrator and turn patties over. Heat for 1-2 more hours.

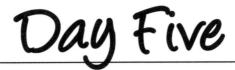

LUNCH:
Veggie Burritos

VEGGIE BURRITOS
Use Garden of Eatin' organic whole wheat burrito shells and stuff with any or all of the following:

green leaf lettuce spinach
diced peppers shredded carrots
homemade ranch dressing
shredded cheese substitute *(optional)*

chopped onions chopped tomatoes
vegetarian refried beans
salsa sliced olives
diced cucumbers

DINNER:
Raw Loaf, Garden Salad,
Tiny Lima Beans *(frozen, prepared according to package directions)*

RAW LOAF*
1 cup almonds, finely ground
1 clove minced garlic
1 rib celery, chopped
1/4 red pepper, chopped
2 Tbsp parsley
2 pitted dates, chopped

1 cup sunflower seeds, ground
2 carrots, finely chopped
1/2 onion, chopped
1/4 yellow pepper, chopped
1/2 tsp Celtic Sea Salt

It is best to soak then rinse the almonds and seeds for 8 hours. A food processor works great to process all of the ingredients for this loaf. Put in glass loaf pan and top with organic ketchup or tomato sauce. Dehydrate at 105 degrees for 4 hours.

*NOTE: This recipe has been adapted from the Celebration Loaf recipe as found in Warming Up to Living Foods by Elysa Markowitz.

Notes: _____

_____

_____

_____

_____

_____

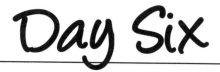

LUNCH:
Spaghetti *(All-raw)*,
Spinach Salad #1 *(See Week One, Day Three, Dinner)*

SPAGHETTI
Pasta—In a bowl add:
2 large zucchinis, which have been peeled and then grated in food processor
1/2 cup chopped mushrooms, use your favorite
6 Italian olives, pitted and halved

Sauce—In a blender, add:

2 cloves garlic   2 vine-ripened tomatoes
1/4 cup sun dried tomatoes*   2 Tbsp extra virgin cold-pressed olive oil
1/4 cup fresh basil   1/4 cup fresh oregano
1 tsp sea salt

Blend well and pour over zucchini.

*Sun Dried Tomatoes—In a large bowl, add:

10 Roma tomatoes, thinly sliced   1/2 cup extra virgin cold-pressed olive oil
3 garlic cloves, minced   1 tsp onion powder
1 tsp sea salt

Marinate for at least 30 minutes. Place on Teflex sheets and dehydrate for 5 hours. Remove from Teflex sheet; turn over onto mesh dehydrator tray and dehydrate for another 5 hours. They should be chewy, not crunchy.

*This all-raw recipe was taken from the book How We All Went Raw by Charles, Coralanne and George Nungesser. Used by permission. Available from Hallelujah Acres (1-800-915-9355).

DINNER:
Garden Salad *(See Week One, Day One, Lunch)*,
Rice and Lightly Steamed Vegetables, Apple Pie Salad

RICE AND LIGHTLY STEAMED VEGETABLES
To prepare brown or basmati rice, boil 2 cups of pure water and 1 teaspoon Celtic Sea Salt. Add 1-1/3 cups of rice, reduce heat, and simmer for 30 minutes without lifting the lid. Remove from stove and let sit for 15 minutes. Fluff with fork.

Lightly steam the following:

2 packages broccoli/cauliflower/carrot mix   1/2 cup onions, chopped
1/2 cup red pepper, chopped   1 tsp parsley
2 cloves garlic, minced

Serve vegetables over rice.

Day Six

APPLE PIE SALAD

4 apples, diced
1/2 cup sliced almonds
1 tsp cinnamon
1/2 tsp allspice
1/4 cup pure maple syrup

1/2 cup organic raisins
1/2 cup organic oatmeal
1/2 tsp Celtic Sea Salt
1 tsp lemon juice

Serve as a salad or spoon onto the following nut crust for a raw apple cobbler.

RAW NUTTY CRUST:

2 cups walnuts
5 organic Medjool dates
1/2 tsp Frontier vanilla

Blend in food processor and pat in square pan.

Notes: _____

_____

_____

_____

_____

_____

_____

_____

_____

_____

_____

_____

_____

_____

Day Seven

LUNCH:
Fruit Plate

FRUIT PLATE

Include such fruits as apple slices, orange sections, banana, red grapes, sliced kiwi, sliced peaches, strawberries, blueberries, raspberries, etc. Don't mix melons with any other fruit as they digest more quickly than other fruits.

DINNER:
Garden Salad *(See Week One, Day One, Lunch)*
Country Vegetable Plate

COUNTRY VEGETABLE PLATE

Choose 3 vegetables from the following suggestions:

Steamed Cabbage - Cut up cabbage. Add small amount of pure water to pot. *(Waterless cookware is excellent for this!)* Add 1/2 to 1 teaspoon of sea salt and 1 tablespoon of olive or grapeseed oil. Cook on low heat until tender.

Fresh Green Beans - Snap beans and rinse. Add beans and 1/2 to 1 teaspoon of sea salt and 1 tablespoon of olive oil to pot. Cook on low heat in small amount of pure water until tender.

New Potatoes - Scrub small new potatoes. Use enough water to just cover potatoes. Add 1/2 to 1 teaspoon of sea salt. Cook on low heat until tender. Drain and add butter blend or Earth Balance to taste.

Summer Squash - Cut up squash into bite-size pieces. Add to large skillet with 1/2 cup pure water, 1/2 to 1 teaspoon of sea salt, 1 tablespoon butter substitute, and 1/2 cup chopped onion. Sauté on low heat until tender.

Steamed Broccoli - Pour about 1-1/2 cups of water in a pot. Place whole broccoli in a steamer basket and place in pot. Bring water to a boil, place lid on pot, and reduce heat. Steam for about 4 minutes. Broccoli should be bright green; pierce stems with a fork to be sure they are tender. Season lightly with sea salt.

Steamed Baby Carrots - Prepare the same way as broccoli.

NOTES:

Holiday Meal

On special occasions, you may find yourself eating more cooked food than usual. Of course, be sure to incorporate any of your favorite fresh, live salads. We recommend extra BarleyMax, fresh juice, and a digestive enzyme with your feast.

HOLIDAY SWEET POTATOES

Peel, cube, and cook 4 sweet potatoes on medium heat in distilled water until tender. Remove potatoes and save water. Put potatoes and 1/3 cup of the water in a large mixing bowl.

Add the following:

1/3 cup raw honey or pure maple syrup
1 tsp Frontier vanilla

3 tbs Earth Balance or butter blend
1/2 cup organic raisins

Blend potatoes, honey, Earth Balance, and vanilla well with your mixer. Add additional water if needed for the potatoes to be soft. Stir in raisins. Spoon into a square baking dish and sprinkle some chopped pecans on top.

CORNBREAD DRESSING

1-1/2 cups corn meal
1 cup chopped green onions
1 Tbsp Rumford baking powder
1/4 cup Vegenaise or almond mayonnaise

3/4 cup chopped celery
1 grated apple
1 cup rice or almond milk

Melt 1-1/2 tablespoons of organic butter in a large pan and bake at 375 degrees until golden brown.

NOTE: Make the cornbread the day before the big feast.

DRESSING

2 cups Imagine No Chicken Broth
2 slices whole-grain bread,
    cut into cubes and toasted
1/2 tsp Celtic Sea Salt

1 tsp marjoram
1/2 tsp thyme
1/2 tsp sage

Mix well and bake at 350 degrees about 45 minutes or until firm.

PEARLED ONIONS and PEAS

Cook according to package directions.

BROCCOLI RICE CASSEROLE

1 small onion, chopped
1/2 tsp Celtic Sea Salt
1 can Amy's Cream of Mushroom Soup
1 rib celery, chopped

2 cups instant brown rice
2 cups distilled water
2 packages chopped broccoli

Steam sauté onion and celery in 2 tablespoons distilled water. Add rice and brown for 5 minutes. Add water and salt. Cover until water is absorbed. Meanwhile, cook broccoli according to package directions. Mix with rice and soup. Pour into a baking dish that has been sprayed with olive oil. Bake at 350 degrees for 25 minutes. Remove from oven and cover with shredded "cheese" *(optional)*. Put lid on so cheese will melt.

CRANBERRY SAUCE

This recipe is taken from Rhonda Malkmus' book,
Recipes for Life from God's Garden.

2 cups fresh or frozen cranberries
1 orange
2 ripe pears
1/2 cup honey
1/4 tsp cinnamon, ginger, and allspice

1/2 cup pitted dates
1 medium delicious apple
1/2 cup raisins
1/4 cup grated orange rind
1/4 cup apple or orange juice

In a food processor, grind cranberries and dates, and transfer to a bowl. Chop peeled orange, apple, and pears and add to bowl. Add raisins, honey, orange rind, juice, and spices. If a gelatin salad is desired, simply increase the apple juice to 1/2 cup and dissolve 4 tablespoons of agar agar for a few minutes, put in a saucepan, and boil for 5 minutes before adding to the salad.

VEGETABLE CASSEROLE

1 small pkg mixed vegetables
3/4 cup Vegenaise
2 tbs Earth Balance or butter blend

1 large pkg broccoli-cauliflower-carrot mix
2 Tbsp Rice Dream milk substitute
1 can water chestnuts, drained and chopped

Cook vegetables together in a small amount of salted *(1 teaspoon)* water. Drain. Mix vegetables, Vegenaise, rice *(or almond)* milk, margarine substitute, and water chestnuts in a bowl. Spray a 9" x 13" dish with olive oil. Pour vegetable mixture in dish. Top with whole grain cracker crumbs and shredded cheese substitute *(optional)*. Cover and bake at 350 degrees for 15-20 minutes or until bubbly.

AMBROSIA

Cut up as many oranges as you want. Add either fresh diced pineapple or canned pineapple, which has been packed in its own juice. Add shredded unsweetened coconut. Stir and allow fruits to marinate for a couple of hours before serving.

DINNER

If you don't want leftovers at night, have a nice garden salad and this wonderful recipe…

PAT'S SPINACH WRAPS

Thaw frozen, chopped spinach. Squeeze dry. Meanwhile sauté chopped onions, diced peppers, and sliced mushrooms just until tender. Remove from heat and add spinach and a little Parmesan Veggie Topping (optional). Stir well, spoon onto a warm whole-wheat tortilla shell, and fold.

Notes: _____

_____

_____

_____

_____

_____

_____

_____

_____

_____

_____

_____

_____

_____

NOTES:

Salad Dressings

There is a wealth of salad dressing ideas in Chapter 16 of *Recipes for Life from God's Garden* by Rhonda Malkmus. She also has a book, *Salad Dressings for Life* with over 117 dressing ideas. Both books can be ordered by calling 1-800-915-9355.

Dr. Joel Robbins suggests a blend of avocado and tomatoes, blended raw tomatoes, or just freshly squeezed lemon juice with a sprinkle of your favorite herbs on your salad. Dr. Joel Fuhrman suggests several low-calorie commercial dressings in his book, *Eat to Live*.

It's best to make salad dressings early in the morning so there are several hours for the dressing to marinate.

NON-DAIRY RANCH DRESSING
1 cup Vegenaise
1 tsp garlic powder
1 Tbsp minced onion
2 tsp lemon juice
1/2 tsp Celtic Sea Salt
3 Tbsp distilled water*

NOTE: If you prefer to use this as a vegetable dip for baby carrots, broccoli florets, cauliflower, sliced squash, sliced cucumbers, celery sticks, etc., then omit the water.

HONEY MUSTARD DRESSING
1/2 cup Westbrae Natural Dijon mustard
4 Tbsp Udo's oil or olive oil
2/3 cup raw honey

Mix dressing well and pour over salad immediately before serving.

SWEET LEMON DRESSING
1/4 cup lemon juice
1 clove garlic, minced
2 Tbsp pure water
1 Tbsp minced onion
1/3 cup raw honey
1/2 tsp crushed basil
pinch of sea salt
1 tsp oregano

Mix dressing well and pour over salad immediately before serving.

AVOCADO DRESSING
1 ripe avocado, mashed
1 freshly-squeezed lemon
herb seasoning to taste

Mix dressing well and pour over salad immediately before serving.

DAISY'S SIMPLE DRESSING
2/3 cup Vegenaise
1/3 cup organic ketchup

Mix dressing well and pour over salad immediately before serving.

Notes: _____

_____

_____

_____

_____

_____

_____

_____

_____

_____

_____

_____

_____

Special Occasion Treats

Most of the following special occasion treats are all-raw; therefore they can be enjoyed often. Most people on the Standard American Diet indulge in sugary desserts *(made with white sugar)* every day of the week.

Again, Rhonda's book contains a chapter of some delightful desserts. Also, most of the Food Show videos have dessert suggestions, too.

FRUIT SMOOTHIE
3 slightly-thawed bananas
6 pitted dates
1 tsp raw honey
2 Tbsp raw almond butter *(optional)*

8 organic strawberries*
1 cup distilled water
1 tsp Frontier vanilla

Start off with only 1 banana, 4 strawberries, and 1/2 cup of water in your blender. Blend until smooth, stop, then add the remainder of the ingredients. Of course, the more water you add, the more like a milkshake it will be. For a creamier smoothie, substitute Rice Dream for the water.

NOTE: Use organic strawberries since regular commercially grown strawberries have been heavily sprayed with pesticides. You can substitute any berries like blueberries or raspberries. You could also make a "chocolate" smoothie by using 5 tablespoons of carob powder in place of the berries and increase the honey to 2 teaspoons. Sprinkle with some chopped walnuts. YUM!

FRUIT SLUSH
Pour 1 cup apple juice, preferably fresh, into your blender. Add 1 cup of frozen organic strawberries. Blend, pour into a pretty glass, add a straw, and sip.

VALDA'S RAW FUDGE
1/4 cup raw sesame seeds
1 cup old fashioned oats
1 cup chopped walnuts

1/4 cup raw sunflower seeds
1 cup chopped pecans

Grind in your food processor then add:
1/2 cup carob powder
1/2 tsp vanilla
2/3 cup raw honey or pure maple syrup

Mix well and pat in an 8-inch square pan that has been sprayed with olive oil. Refrigerate until firm, then cut into squares.

Special Occasion Treats

continued

RAW APPLE PIE
Crust:
1-1/4 cups pecans

5 Medjool dates, pitted

3 Tbsp pure maple syrup

1 cup walnuts

1/4 tsp sea salt

1 tsp Frontier vanilla

Process using the 'S' blade on your food processor; then pat in a pie plate.

Filling:
2 Granny Smith apples

1/2 cup organic raisins

1/4 cup raw honey

1 tsp cinnamon

1 tsp fresh lemon juice

2 Fuji or Cameo apples

1/4 tsp Celtic Sea Salt

4 Medjool dates, pitted

1 Tbsp ground flaxseed

Peel 1 Granny Smith and 1 sweet apple. Using the S-blade, process the apples and dates into small chunks. Transfer to another bowl and add ground flaxseed, salt, honey, cinnamon, lemon juice, and raisins. Stir well. Coarsely chop the last 2 apples. Add to mixture, stir, and pour onto crust. Top with chopped nuts. Refrigerate.

HOLIDAY RAW SWEET POTATO PIE
Crust:
1 pound pitted dates

1 cup ground almonds

Process dates and ground almonds in food processor using the S-blade until the mixture pulls away from the sides to form a ball. Press into pie plate with wet fingers to form a crust. Add filling.

Filling:
3 medium sweet potatoes
   (peeled and cut into chunks)

1/4 cup unsweetened coconut

1 tsp fresh lemon juice

2-3 oz ground walnuts

6 pitted dates

1/3 cup organic honey

3/4 tsp nutmeg

1-1/2 tsp cinnamon

Run potatoes and dates through your juicer, using the blank. In a bowl, add to the pulped sweet potato/date mixture, the remaining filling ingredients and mix well.

Topping:
2 oz ground walnuts

Refrigerate and enjoy. Makes two 8-inch pies.

Special Occasion Treats

continued

VERY STRAWBERRY PIE
Crust:

1 cup almonds
10 Medjool dates, pitted

1/2 tsp vanilla
2 tsp raw honey or maple syrup

Process the above ingredients in your food processor using the 'S' blade, then pat in a pie plate.

Filling:

4 cups organic strawberries
1 banana
4 tsp ground flaxseed

10 Medjool dates, pitted
2 tsp lemon juice

Process 2 cups of strawberries, dates, banana, lemon juice, and flaxseed until smooth. Chop remainder of strawberries and add to mixture. Stir well and pour onto crust. Garnish with sliced strawberries. Refrigerate.

BANANA OATMEAL DROP COOKIES

3 large bananas
2 cups rolled oats
1 tsp vanilla
2 tsp raw honey

1/3 cup grapeseed or olive oil
1 cup chopped Medjool dates
1/2 cup chopped walnuts
1/8 tsp sea salt

Preheat oven to 350 degrees. Combine all ingredients. Allow to rest 15 minutes to let the flavors mingle. Drop by teaspoonfuls onto a sheet lightly sprayed with olive oil. Bake for 20 minutes.

ALMOND BUTTER BALLS

1/2 cup almond butter
1 cup old fashioned oats
1/4 cup chopped pecans

1/2 cup raw honey
1/2 tsp almond extract

Form into balls and roll in additional chopped pecans. Refrigerate.

BANANA-STRAWBERRY "ICE CREAM"

Alternate running frozen bananas and frozen organic strawberries through your Champion or Green Star Juicer with the blank in place. You can add a little honey to sweeten if needed.

VALDA'S YUMMY PERSIMMON ICE CREAM

3-1/2 cups almond milk
1-1/2 cups persimmon pulp *(whole persimmons that have been pureed)*

1/2 cup honey
1 tsp Frontier vanilla
3/4 cup chopped pecans

Dissolve honey in almond milk almond milk. Stir in vanilla, persimmon pulp, and pecans. Pour in 1/2-gallon ice cream freezer and freeze.

STRAWBERRY SHAKE

1 cup rice or almond milk
2 frozen bananas
5-6 frozen organic strawberries

Blend and enjoy.

BUCKWHEATIE BARS

(Taken from Serene Allison's all-raw book, *Rejuvenate Your Life: Recipes for Energy*. (Used by permission.)

The base for this recipe is Buckwheaties. To make them just sprout buckwheat groats for 2 days. Pour 2-1/3 cups of buckwheat groats into a large bowl and soak overnight with plenty of distilled water. The next morning pour the groats into a large colander. Rinse them well and run them halfway up the sides of the colander using your fingers. Place colander on a plate and cover with a towel. Rinse at night and in the morning for 2 days. Then place the sprouts on mesh dehydrator trays and dehydrate at 105 degrees until thoroughly dry.

In a bowl mix the following:

4 cups of buckwheaties
1 cup raw honey
1/2–3/4 cup tahini or raw almond butter
3/4 cup golden flaxseed meal *(grind in coffee grinder)*

Add goodies to your heart's content:

A few handfuls of raisins
A few handfuls of chopped dates
A few handfuls of chopped unsulfured apricots
A few handfuls of chopped walnuts and/or almonds

You could also add some handfuls of pumpkin seeds, sunflower seeds, and whole flax seeds. Optional—try goji berries or pine nuts.

Mix all together. If it seems too dry and crumbly, add a little more tahini/almond butter, honey, and/or flax meal to bind. Put in a pie plate sprayed with oil and refrigerate. When firm, cut into bars. These freeze well.

Special Occasion Treats

HEDGEHOG BALLS

1 cup pitted dates
1 cup raw almonds
1 cup shredded *(unsweetened)* coconut
2 tsp vanilla extract
2 Tbsp raw honey extract

1 cup organic raisins
2 cups rolled oats
2 Tbsp raw carob
1/2 tsp peppermint

Place dates and raisins in food processor and blend into small pieces. Add the almonds, oats, coconut, and carob powder. Blend until the mixture resembles breadcrumbs. Add the extracts and honey. Stop the machine and check if the texture is correct by taking a small amount into the palm of your hand and roll into a ball. If the mixture does not bind, add extra honey or some apple juice.

APPLE LEMONADE

Juice 8-10 Fuji or Gala apples in a Champion or Green Star Juicer. Then juice 1/2 of an organic lemon, including the peel. Refrigerate until cold and serve with a lemon slice. For pink lemonade, add 1/8 teaspoon of BeetMax from Hallelujah Acres.

ALMOND COOKIES (Taken from Rhonda Malkmus' book *Recipes for Life from God's Garden*)

2 cups almonds
1/2 cup unfiltered honey
unsweetened coconut

Grind almonds into a fine meal. Work in enough honey to make a sticky dough. Roll into balls or log-shape and roll in coconut. Chill then slice.

YUMMY PEACH COBBLER

5 cups sliced peaches
3 Tbsp pure maple syrup
3 Tbsp unbleached, unenriched flour

1/2 cup all-fruit apricot preserves
1/8 tsp nutmeg

Mix the above ingredients well. Pour into a square pan and bake for 20 minutes at 350 degrees.

Topping:

1-1/2 cups organic oats
4 Tbsp pure maple syrup
1/4 tsp sea salt

4 Tbsp unbleached flour
1 tsp vanilla

Mix and spoon over baked filling. Bake for 15 additional minutes. Serve warm.

Special Occasion Treats

continued

FRUIT SOUP

2 cups sliced grapes	1-1/2 cups blueberries
1 cup diced strawberries	1 cup diced pineapple

Add 2 cups organic apple juice and 1 cup of freshly squeezed orange juice. Stir gently. Cover bowl tightly and refrigerate until ready to serve.

MARY LYNN'S MEXICAN PINWHEELS
Use organic whole-wheat tortilla shells and layer the following:
1. Rice cream cheese
2. Warmed organic refried beans
3. Chopped onions, black olives, spinach, onions, or any vegetables you like
4. Grated cheese substitute

Roll up and cut into 1-1/2 inch pieces.

NOTE: For Italian Pinwheels, just substitute organic spaghetti sauce for the refried beans.

Notes: _____

_____

_____

_____

_____

_____

_____

_____

_____

_____

_____

_____

Helpful Tips

1. If you are unable to juice vegetables, try CarrotJuiceMax.

2. Never drink carbonated drinks because an average 12-oz cola contains 150 calories and has over 9 teaspoons of sugar per can! Soft drinks are very acidic and will cause the body to rob calcium, which is alkaline, from the bones and teeth in order to neutralize the high acid.

3. Never use a microwave oven because microwaving results in more lost nutrients than any other heating method. It also changes the molecular structure of food.

4. Nutritional yeast is 50% protein and a good source of several B vitamins. It gives a cheesy flavor to your recipes.

5. Lemon juice can be substituted for vinegar in salad dressing recipes.

6. Did you know that aluminum has an affinity for the brain? Use Rumford aluminum-free baking powder. Avoid aluminum cookware and also deodorants that contain aluminum.

7. According to Dr. T Colin Campbell in his book *The China Project*, "animal protein raises blood cholesterol—a major risk factor for heart disease—more than does the much more feared saturated fat. This means that, in effect, lean meats may be just as damaging to your cholesterol levels as that piece of bacon you've been avoiding."

8. Canola oil should be avoided! It comes from the rape seed plant, which is actually a weed and the most toxic of all food-oil plants.

9. When buying dried fruits and vegetables, look for those that are organic and do not contain sulfur dioxide, a harmful preservative.

10. Remember, fresh is always best; frozen would be the next best purchase. When buying canned foods, always look for those that are organic and have lined cans.

11. Did you know that some syrup producers might inject a maple tree with formaldehyde, a known carcinogen, to prolong the sap flow? This is a good reason to buy organic maple syrup!

12. Got the munchies? Try drinking a cup of pure water. Wait five minutes; if you are still hungry then mix up some trail mix. Pour some raw sunflower seeds, raw nuts, organic raisins, and dried cherries in a bag. Shake and eat one handful.

Index

MOSTLY RAW FOODS

COOKED FOODS

Index

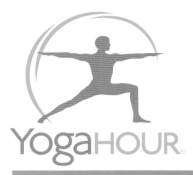

YogaHOUR

Syllabus & Sequences Volume 1

yogahour® (yH): an accessible, affordable, expertly taught flow/form class that offers clear and specific alignment instructions for the fit beginner. yH seeks to help support and sustain the local studio and longevity of practice.

The key to effective sequencing is a balance between **consistency** and **creativity.** All of the yH sequences share similarities (consistency). All of them share distinct differences (creativity). yH classes are designed to offer a well rounded and balanced class (consistency). Although one pose does indeed lead to another, none of these sequences are built around or geared toward a particular pose. And yet, all of these sequences can easily be modified (creativity).

What makes the yH syllabus the yH syllabus? Why this pose and not that pose? The aim of the yH syllabus is to minimize risk and maximize reward in a flow/form class setting geared toward the fit beginner (students without any major limitations or injuries). Alignment itself is the primary agent that minimizes risk and maximizes reward. For a complete description of how to get into and out of every one of these poses, please refer to the manual *Yogahour®: Inform Your Flow* (SSR) by Darren Rhodes.

yogahour® barefoot bootcamp is all about syllabus as sequence. Barefoot bootcamp is a dharma difficult yet doable challenge that is sure to make an imprint on your practice. The poses from the yogahour syllabus are broken into categories: Standing + Supine, Arm Balances, Backbends, & Forward Folds including a set Warm Up and a set Cool Down Sequence.

Yogahour® founder, author, and creator of this project: Darren Rhodes: www.YogaOasis.com

Sequence Designers and Models:
Darren Rhodes: www.YogaOasis.com
Brigette Finley: www.YogaOasis.com
Alexis Finley: www.YogaOasis.com
Sam Rice: www.SamRiceYoga.com
Ellen Niedringhaus: www.BlueBirdYoga.com
Beth Daunis: www.BethDaunis.com

Design: Mackie Osborne, Milo Longstaff, Joanne Miller
Editors: Joanne Miller, Shawn Asplundh, Bre Downing, Christine Reitmayr
Photographer for Darren Rhodes, Sam Rice, and Beth Daunis: Jade Beall www.JadeBeall.com
Printed in China by Prolong Press Limited

sequence 1 with Darren Rhodes

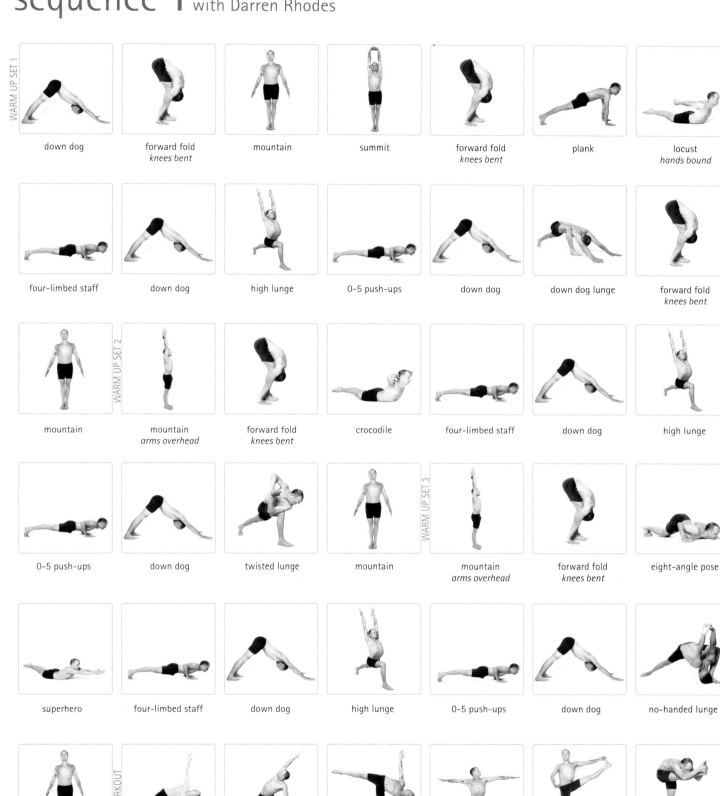

WARM UP SET 1

| down dog | forward fold *knees bent* | mountain | summit | forward fold *knees bent* | plank | locust *hands bound* |

| four-limbed staff | down dog | high lunge | 0-5 push-ups | down dog | down dog lunge | forward fold *knees bent* |

WARM UP SET 2

| mountain | mountain *arms overhead* | forward fold *knees bent* | crocodile | four-limbed staff | down dog | high lunge |

| 0-5 push-ups | down dog | twisted lunge | mountain | mountain *arms overhead* | forward fold *knees bent* | eight-angle pose |

WARM UP SET 3

| superhero | four-limbed staff | down dog | high lunge | 0-5 push-ups | down dog | no-handed lunge |

WORKOUT

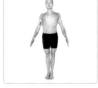
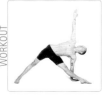
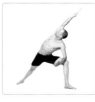

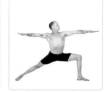
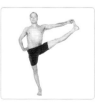
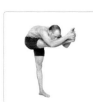

| mountain | triangle | extended side angle *forearm to knee* | half moon | warrior 2 | standing sage 2 | bowing sage |

sequence 1 with Darren Rhodes

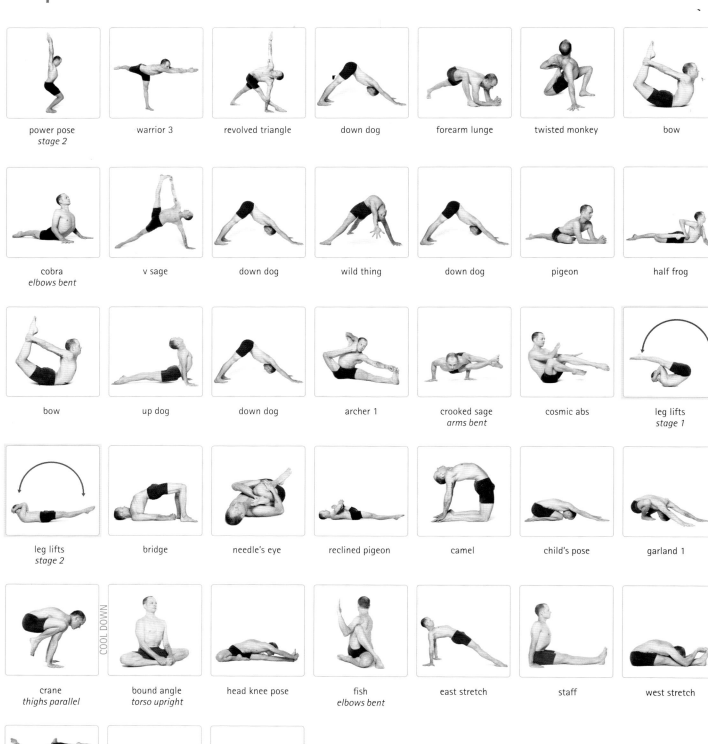

power pose *stage 2*	warrior 3
revolved triangle	down dog
forearm lunge	twisted monkey
bow	

cobra *elbows bent* · v sage · down dog · wild thing · down dog · pigeon · half frog

bow · up dog · down dog · archer 1 · crooked sage *arms bent* · cosmic abs · leg lifts *stage 1*

leg lifts *stage 2* · bridge · needle's eye · reclined pigeon · camel · child's pose · garland 1

COOL DOWN

crane *thighs parallel* · bound angle *torso upright* · head knee pose · fish *elbows bent* · east stretch · staff · west stretch

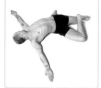

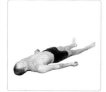

double diamond · reclined child's pose · pose of repose

sequence 2 with Darren Rhodes

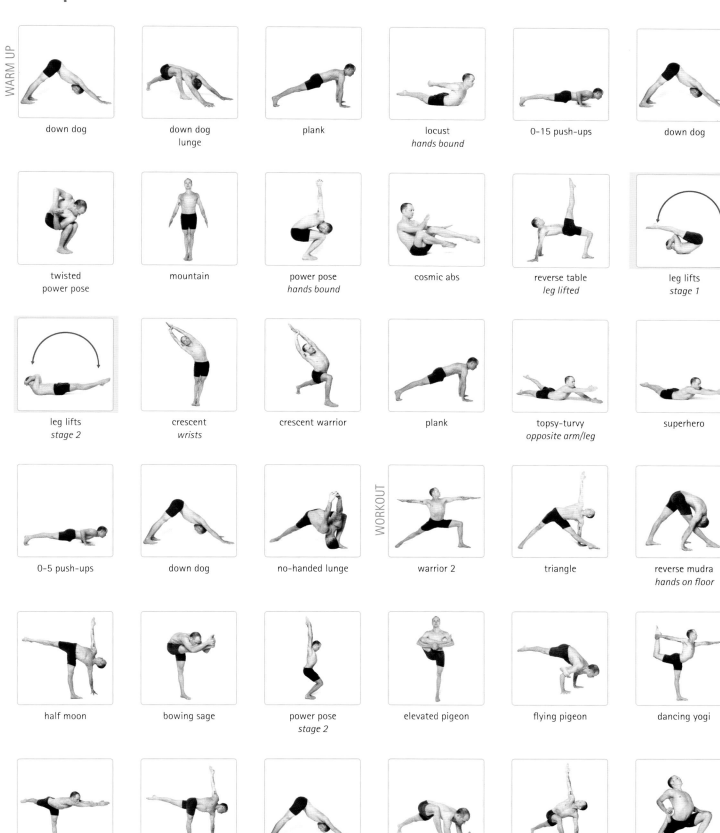

WARM UP

down dog	down dog lunge	plank	locust *hands bound*	0-15 push-ups	down dog
twisted power pose	mountain	power pose *hands bound*	cosmic abs	reverse table *leg lifted*	leg lifts *stage 1*
leg lifts *stage 2*	crescent *wrists*	crescent warrior	plank	topsy-turvy *opposite arm/leg*	superhero

WORKOUT

0-5 push-ups	down dog	no-handed lunge	warrior 2	triangle	reverse mudra *hands on floor*
half moon	bowing sage	power pose *stage 2*	elevated pigeon	flying pigeon	dancing yogi
warrior 3	revolved half moon	down dog	forearm lunge	revolved lunge	monkey lunge *quad stretch*

sequence 2 with Darren Rhodes

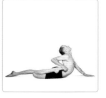

elevated
half frog

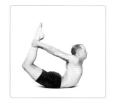

bow

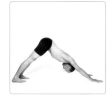

down dog

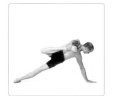

baby bird

COOL DOWN

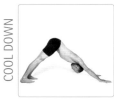

down dog

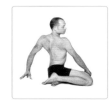

twisted sage
stage 1

east stretch

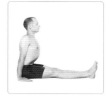

staff

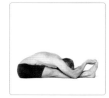

west stretch

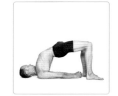

bridge

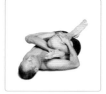

needle's eye

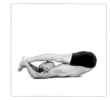

reclined west stretch

double diamond

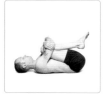

reclined child's pose

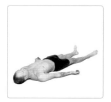

pose of repose

sequence 3 with Darren Rhodes

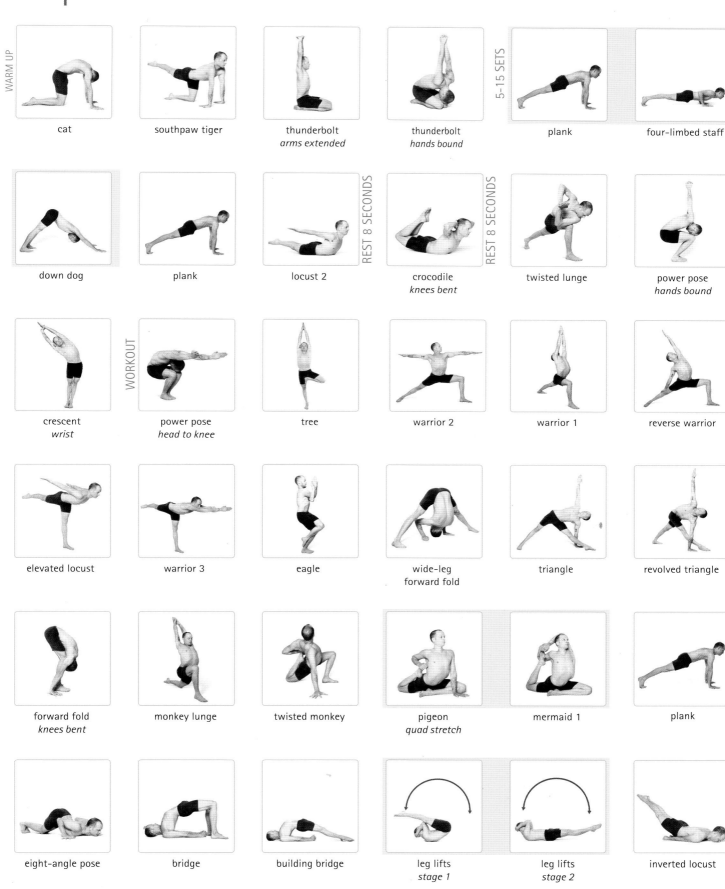

WARM UP

cat

southpaw tiger

thunderbolt
arms extended

thunderbolt
hands bound

5-15 SETS

plank

four-limbed staff

down dog

plank

locust 2

REST 8 SECONDS

crocodile
knees bent

REST 8 SECONDS

twisted lunge

power pose
hands bound

WORKOUT

crescent
wrist

power pose
head to knee

tree

warrior 2

warrior 1

reverse warrior

elevated locust

warrior 3

eagle

wide-leg
forward fold

triangle

revolved triangle

forward fold
knees bent

monkey lunge

twisted monkey

pigeon
quad stretch

mermaid 1

plank

eight-angle pose

bridge

building bridge

leg lifts
stage 1

leg lifts
stage 2

inverted locust

sequence 3 with Darren Rhodes

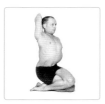

cow face 2

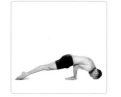

peacock
head on floor

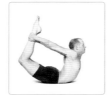

bow

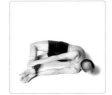

sideways bow

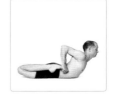

frog

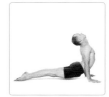

up dog

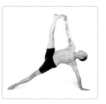

v sage

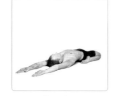

reclined hero

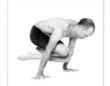

tremulous

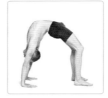

upward bow

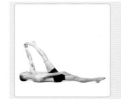

reclined big toe

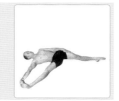

reclined big toe
leg to side

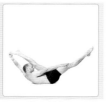

reclined big toe
forehead to knee,
foot off floor

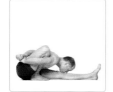

m sage 1

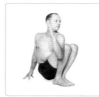

noose
elbow bent

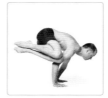

turned crane

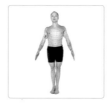

mountain

COOL DOWN

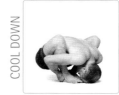

garland 2

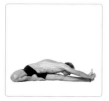

head knee pose

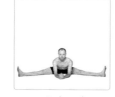

seated angle

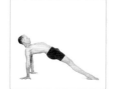

east stretch

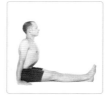

staff

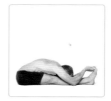

west stretch

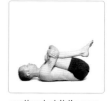

reclined child's pose

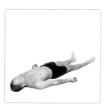

pose of repose

sequence 4 with Darren Rhodes

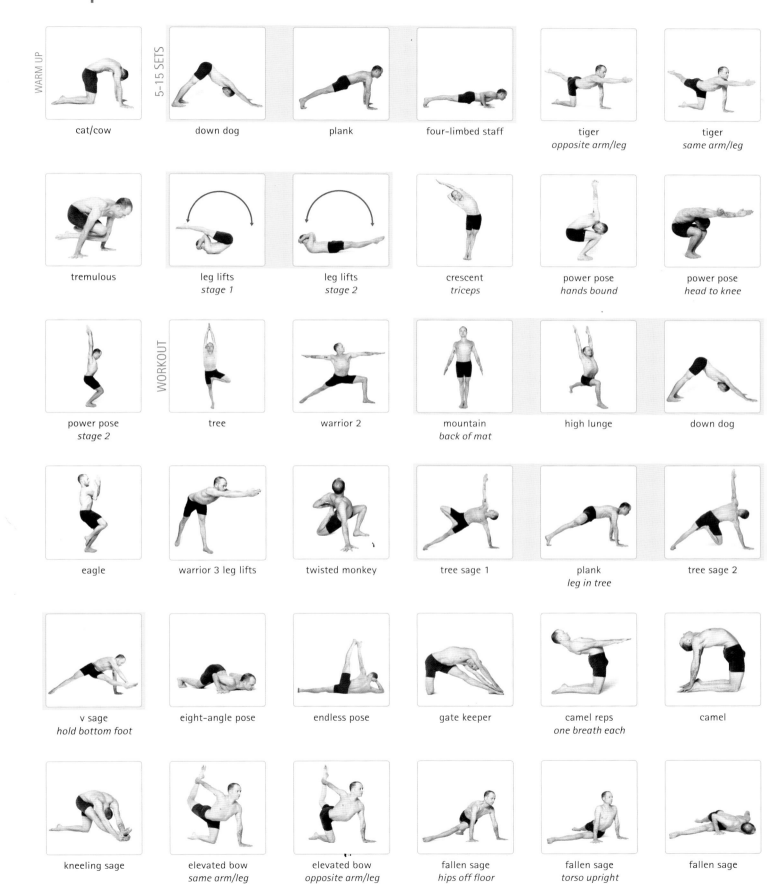

WARM UP

cat/cow

5-15 SETS

down dog

plank

four-limbed staff

tiger
opposite arm/leg

tiger
same arm/leg

tremulous

leg lifts
stage 1

leg lifts
stage 2

crescent
triceps

power pose
hands bound

power pose
head to knee

WORKOUT

power pose
stage 2

tree

warrior 2

mountain
back of mat

high lunge

down dog

eagle

warrior 3 leg lifts

twisted monkey

tree sage 1

plank
leg in tree

tree sage 2

v sage
hold bottom foot

eight-angle pose

endless pose

gate keeper

camel reps
one breath each

camel

kneeling sage

elevated bow
same arm/leg

elevated bow
opposite arm/leg

fallen sage
hips off floor

fallen sage
torso upright

fallen sage

sequence 4 with Darren Rhodes

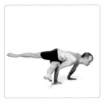

k sage 1

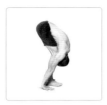

forward fold
knees bent

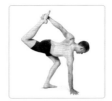

revolved sugar cane

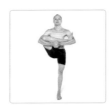

elevated pigeon

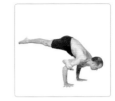

flying pigeon

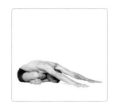

fire logs

bridge

5 SHORT SETS

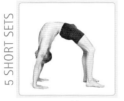

upward bow

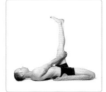

Tibetan weaponry 1

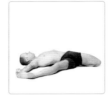

Tibetan weaponry 2

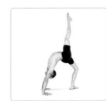

upward bow
leg lifted

COOL DOWN

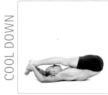

reclined west stretch

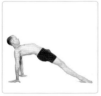

east stretch

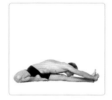

head knee pose

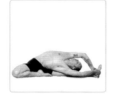

revolved
head knee pose

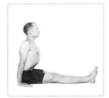

staff

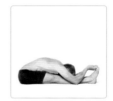

west stretch

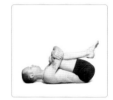

reclined
child's pose

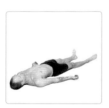

pose of repose

sequence 5 with Darren Rhodes

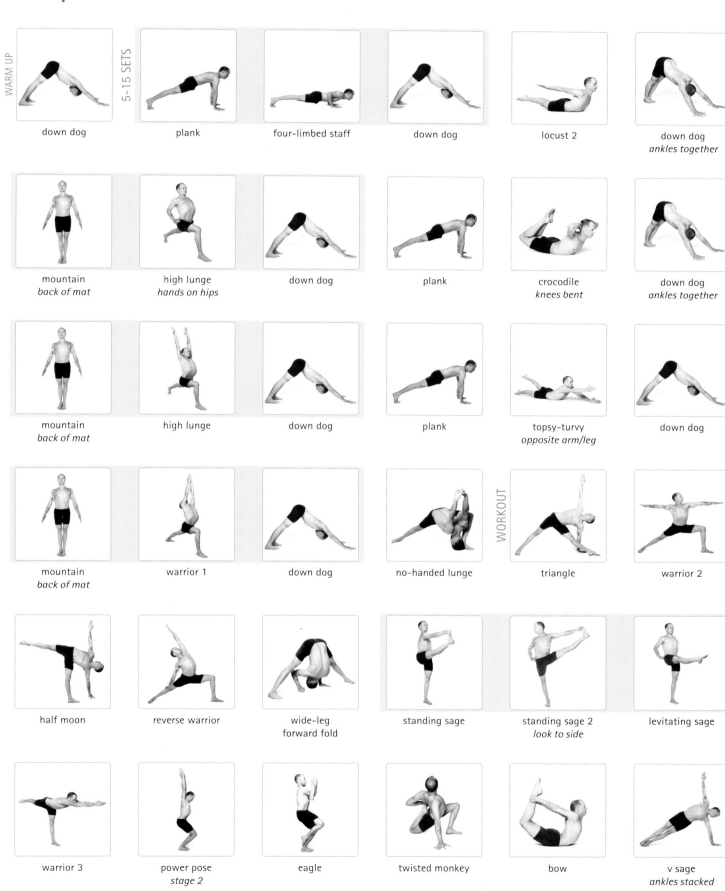

WARM UP

down dog

5-15 SETS

plank

four-limbed staff

down dog

locust 2

down dog
ankles together

mountain
back of mat

high lunge
hands on hips

down dog

plank

crocodile
knees bent

down dog
ankles together

mountain
back of mat

high lunge

down dog

plank

topsy-turvy
opposite arm/leg

down dog

mountain
back of mat

warrior 1

down dog

no-handed lunge

WORKOUT

triangle

warrior 2

half moon

reverse warrior

wide-leg
forward fold

standing sage

standing sage 2
look to side

levitating sage

warrior 3

power pose
stage 2

eagle

twisted monkey

bow

v sage
ankles stacked

sequence 5 with Darren Rhodes

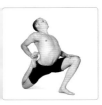
monkey lunge
quad stretch

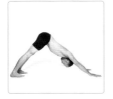
down dog

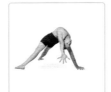
wild thing

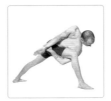
bound side angle

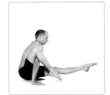
one-hand
arm pose

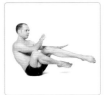
cosmic abs

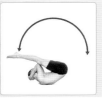
leg lifts
stage 1

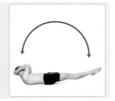
leg lifts
stage 2

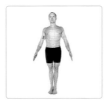
mountain

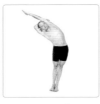
crescent
triceps

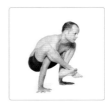
arm pressure pose

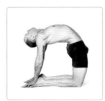
camel

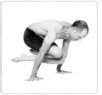
tremulous

upward bow

COOL DOWN

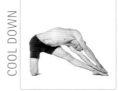
gate keeper

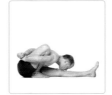
m sage 1

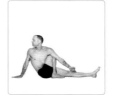
m sage 3
hand to floor

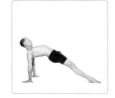
east stretch

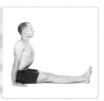
staff

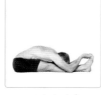
west stretch

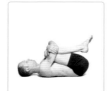
reclined child's pose

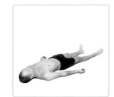
pose of repose

sequence 6 with Brigette Finley

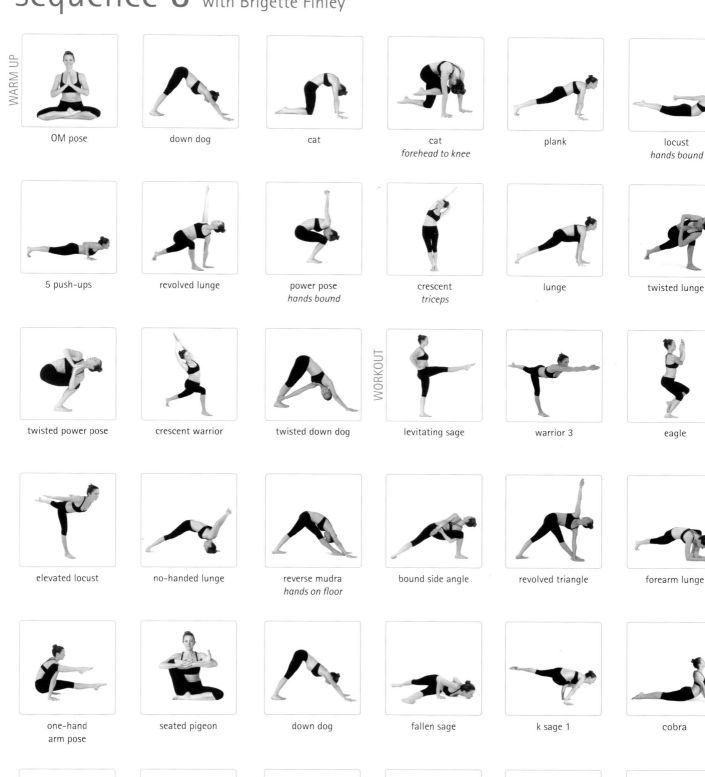

WARM UP

OM pose	down dog	cat	cat *forehead to knee*	plank	locust *hands bound*
5 push-ups	revolved lunge	power pose *hands bound*	crescent *triceps*	lunge	twisted lunge
twisted power pose	crescent warrior	twisted down dog	levitating sage	warrior 3	eagle
elevated locust	no-handed lunge	reverse mudra *hands on floor*	bound side angle	revolved triangle	forearm lunge
one-hand arm pose	seated pigeon	down dog	fallen sage	k sage 1	cobra

WORKOUT

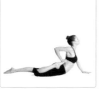
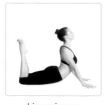

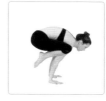
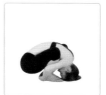
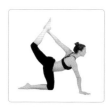

elevated half frog	king pigeon *shins vertical*	bow *hands to ankles*	crane	garland 2	elevated bow *opposite arm/leg*

sequence 6 with Brigette Finley

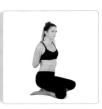

cow face 2

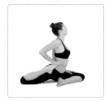

pigeon
quad stretch

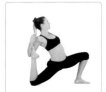

mermaid 2

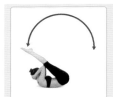

leg lifts
stage 1

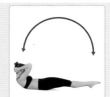

leg lifts
stage 2

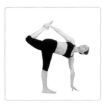

revolved sugar cane

arm pressure pose

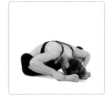

star

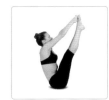

both big toes pose

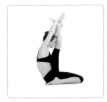

heron

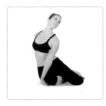

twisted sage

upward bow

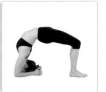

inverted staff

COOL DOWN

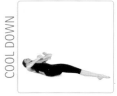

reclined pigeon

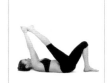

reclined bowing sage

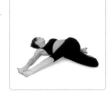

Tibetan weaponry 3

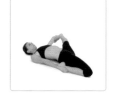

Tibetan weaponry 2

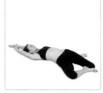

double diamond

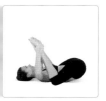

happy baby

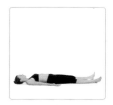

pose of repose

sequence 7 with Alexis Finley

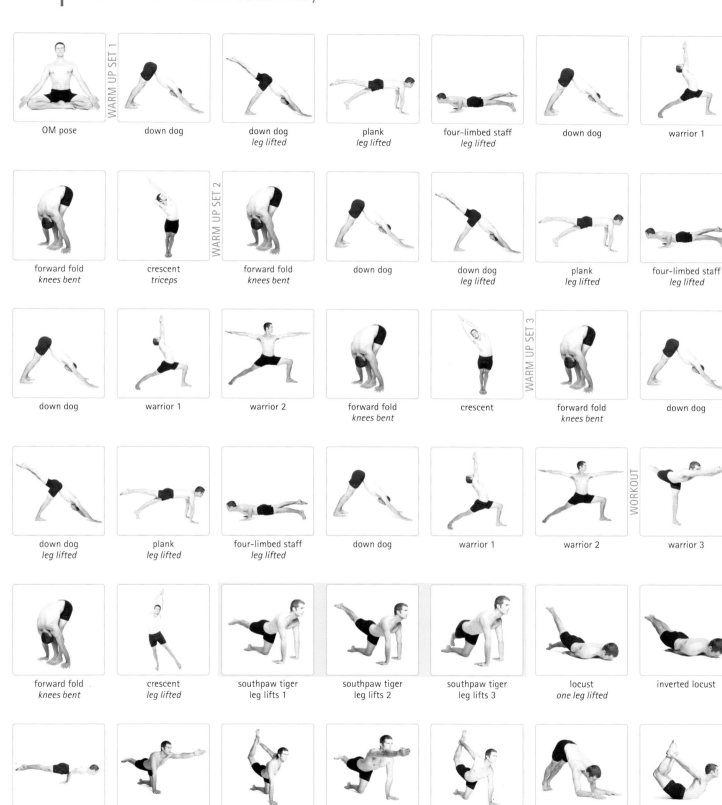

WARM UP SET 1

OM pose

down dog

down dog
leg lifted

plank
leg lifted

four-limbed staff
leg lifted

down dog

warrior 1

WARM UP SET 2

forward fold
knees bent

crescent
triceps

forward fold
knees bent

down dog

down dog
leg lifted

plank
leg lifted

four-limbed staff
leg lifted

WARM UP SET 3

down dog

warrior 1

warrior 2

forward fold
knees bent

crescent

forward fold
knees bent

down dog

WORKOUT

down dog
leg lifted

plank
leg lifted

four-limbed staff
leg lifted

down dog

warrior 1

warrior 2

warrior 3

forward fold
knees bent

crescent
leg lifted

southpaw tiger
leg lifts 1

southpaw tiger
leg lifts 2

southpaw tiger
leg lifts 3

locust
one leg lifted

inverted locust

peacock

tiger
opposite arm/leg

elevated bow
opposite arm/leg

tiger
same arm/leg

elevated bow
same arm/leg

dolphin

bow
thighs up

sequence 7 with Alexis Finley

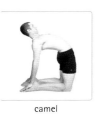
camel

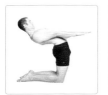
camel
arms parallel

thunderbolt
hands bound

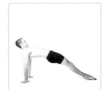
east stretch

warrior 1
eagle arms

eagle

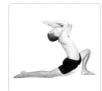
monkey lunge
eagle arms

bound side angle

triangle

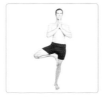
tree

revolved triangle

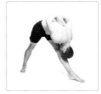
reverse mudra

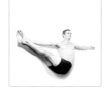
firmly rotated pose

reverse table

reverse table
leg lifted

both-big-toes
pose

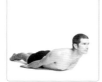
locust 1

lions breath

crane
ankles crossed

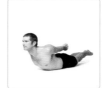
locust
hands bound

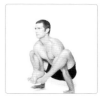
arm pressure pose

bow
thighs down

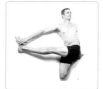
Tibetan weaponry 3

fallen sage
side stretch

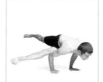
k sage 1

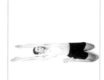
reclined hero

mermaid 2

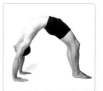
upward bow

double diamond

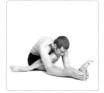
holy cow pose

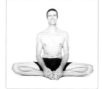
bound angle
torso upright

fire logs
torso upright

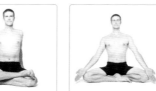
meditation pose
one minute

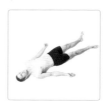
pose of repose

14

sequence 8 with Sam Rice

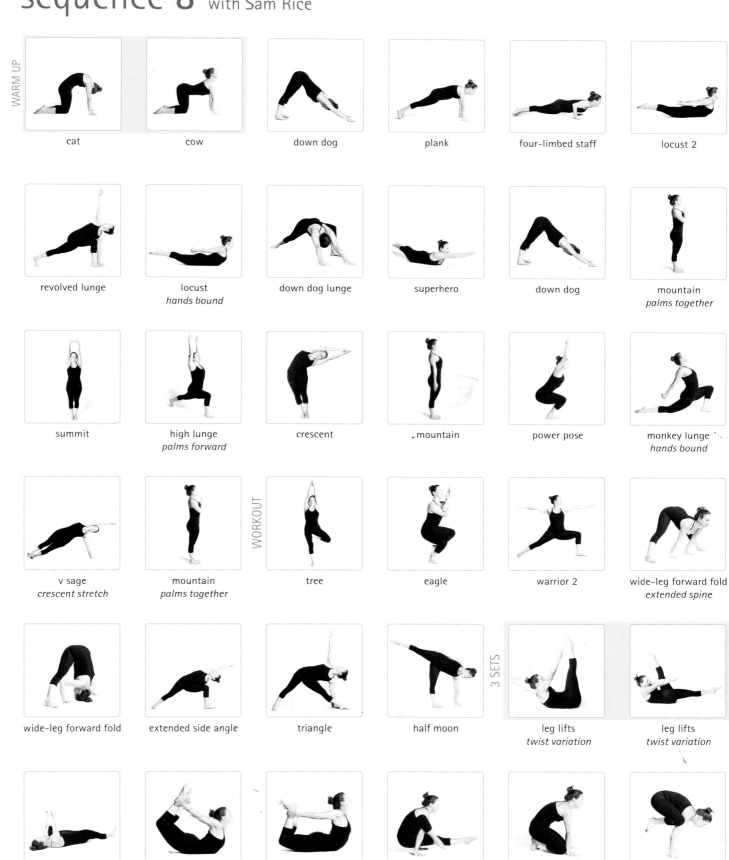

WARM UP

| cat | cow | down dog | plank | four-limbed staff | locust 2 |

| revolved lunge | locust
hands bound | down dog lunge | superhero | down dog | mountain
palms together |

| summit | high lunge
palms forward | crescent | .mountain | power pose | monkey lunge
hands bound |

WORKOUT

| v sage
crescent stretch | mountain
palms together | tree | eagle | warrior 2 | wide-leg forward fold
extended spine |

3 SETS

| wide-leg forward fold | extended side angle | triangle | half moon | leg lifts
twist variation | leg lifts
twist variation |

| reclined lunge | bow | bow
feet flexed | one-hand arm pose | thunderbolt
toe crusher | crane
shins parallel |

15

sequence 8 with Sam Rice

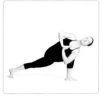
twisted lunge

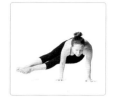
two-leg k sage

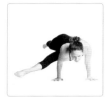
k sage 1

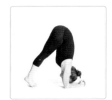
dolphin

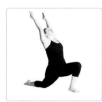
monkey lunge
palms apart

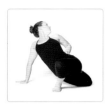
twisted monkey

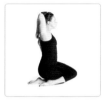
cow face 2

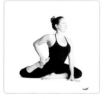
pigeon
quad stretch

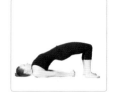
bridge

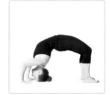
upward bow
head on floor

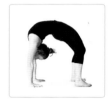
upward bow

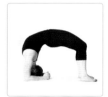
inverted staff

COOL DOWN

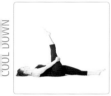
reclined big toe
prep

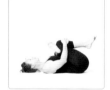
needle's eye

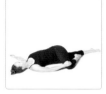
reclined twist

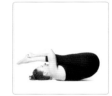
reclined west stretch

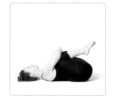
reclined
child's pose

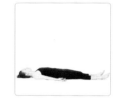
pose of repose

sequence 9 with Ellen Niedringhaus

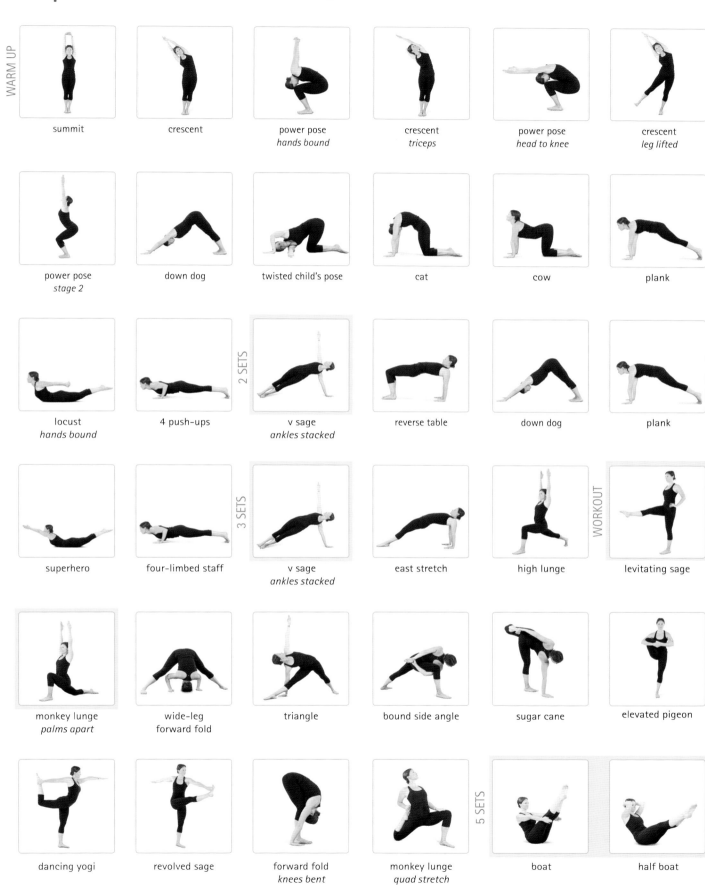

WARM UP

summit

crescent

power pose
hands bound

crescent
triceps

power pose
head to knee

crescent
leg lifted

power pose
stage 2

down dog

twisted child's pose

cat

cow

plank

2 SETS

locust
hands bound

4 push-ups

v sage
ankles stacked

reverse table

down dog

plank

3 SETS

superhero

four-limbed staff

v sage
ankles stacked

east stretch

high lunge

WORKOUT

levitating sage

monkey lunge
palms apart

wide-leg
forward fold

triangle

bound side angle

sugar cane

elevated pigeon

dancing yogi

revolved sage

forward fold
knees bent

monkey lunge
quad stretch

5 SETS

boat

half boat

sequence 9 with Ellen Niedringhaus

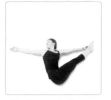

firmly rotated pose

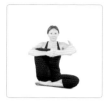

seated pigeon

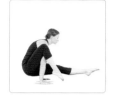

one-hand arm pose

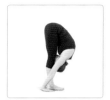

forward fold

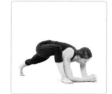

forearm lunge

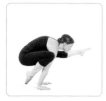

one-leg crane
(b.)

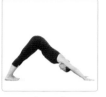

down dog

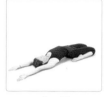

reclined hero

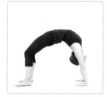

upward bow

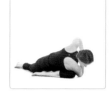

twisted pigeon 1

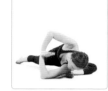

twisted pigeon 2

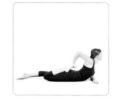

half frog

COOL DOWN

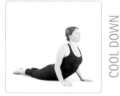

cobra
elbows bent

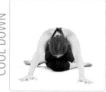

cow face 1
forward fold

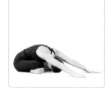

fire logs

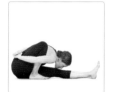

m sage 1

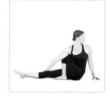

m sage 3
hand to shin

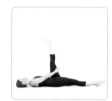

reclined big toe
prep

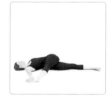

reclined
revolved sage

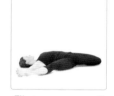

Tibetan weaponry 2

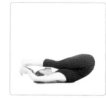

reclined west stretch

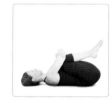

reclined child's pose

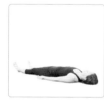

pose of repose

sequence 10 with Darren Rhodes

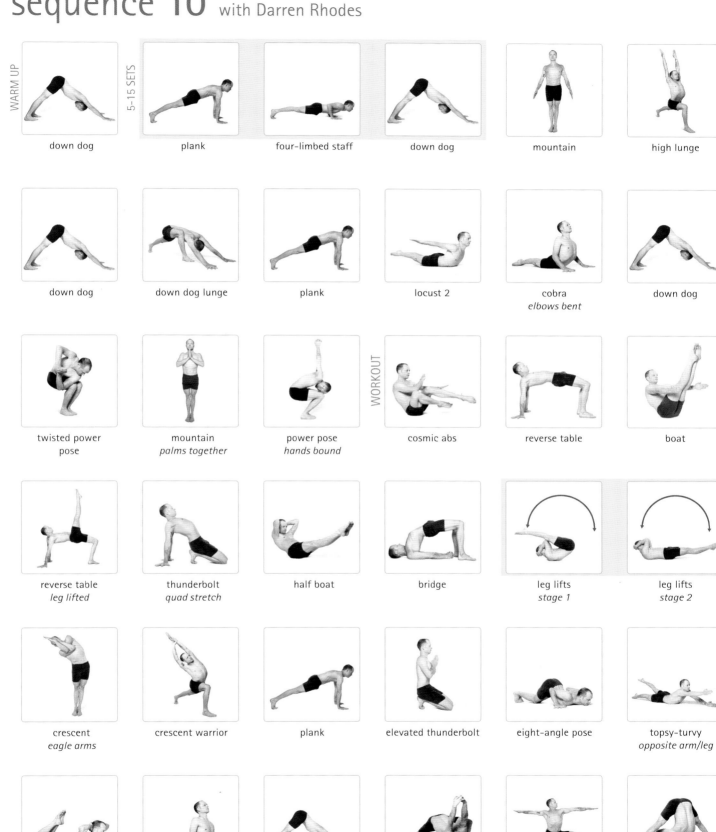

WARM UP

5-15 SETS

down dog | plank | four-limbed staff | down dog | mountain | high lunge

down dog | down dog lunge | plank | locust 2 | cobra *elbows bent* | down dog

twisted power pose | mountain *palms together* | power pose *hands bound* | WORKOUT — cosmic abs | reverse table | boat

reverse table *leg lifted* | thunderbolt *quad stretch* | half boat | bridge | leg lifts *stage 1* | leg lifts *stage 2*

crescent *eagle arms* | crescent warrior | plank | elevated thunderbolt | eight-angle pose | topsy-turvy *opposite arm/leg*

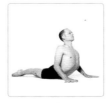
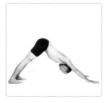
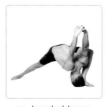
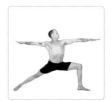
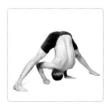

crocodile *knees bent* | cobra *elbows bent* | down dog | no-handed lunge | warrior 2 | wide-leg forward fold

sequence 10 with Darren Rhodes

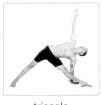
triangle

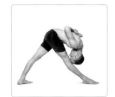
reverse mudra

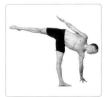
half moon
top arm in mountain

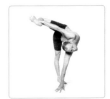
sugar cane

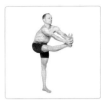
bowing sage
stage 1

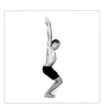
power pose
stage 2

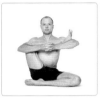
seated pigeon

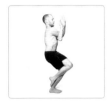
eagle

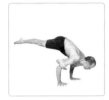
flying pigeon

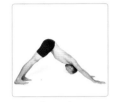
down dog

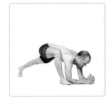
forearm lunge

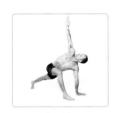
revolved lunge

monkey lunge
quad stretch

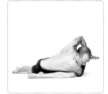
twisted pigeon 1

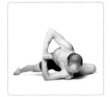
twisted pigeon 2

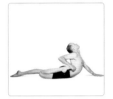
elevated half frog

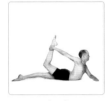
one-leg bow

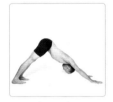
down dog

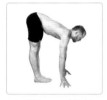
half forward fold

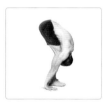
forward fold
knees bent

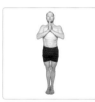
mountain
palms together

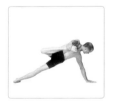
baby bird

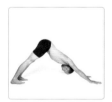
down dog

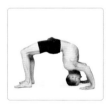
upward bow
head on floor

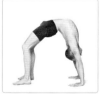
upward bow

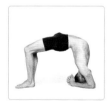
inverted staff

COOL DOWN

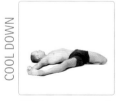
Tibetan weaponry 2

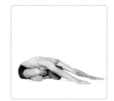
fire logs

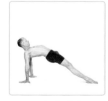
east stretch

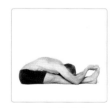
west stretch

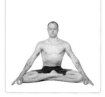
accomplished pose

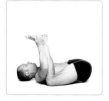
happy baby

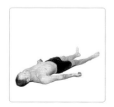
pose of repose

sequence 11 with Darren Rhodes

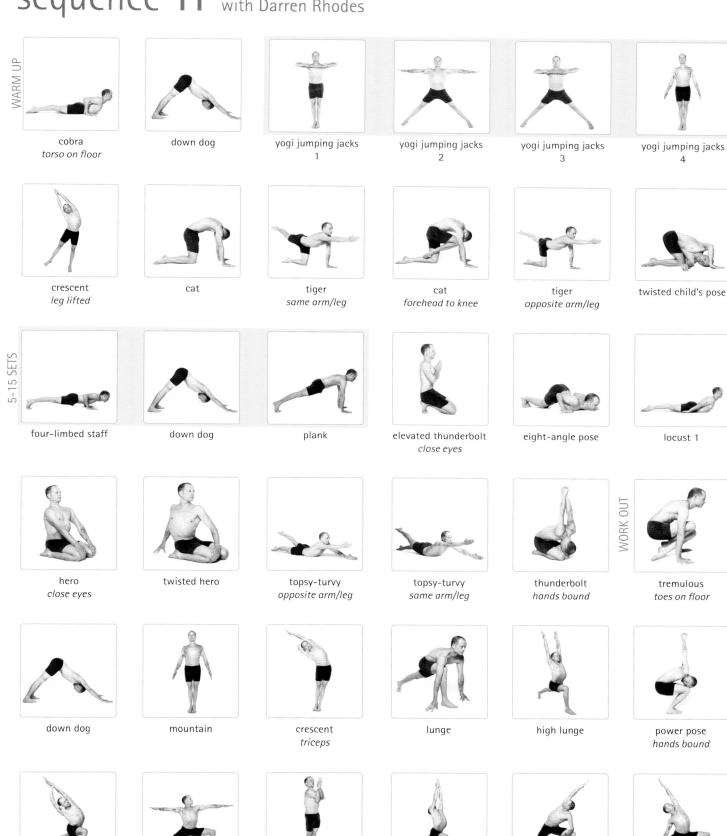

WARM UP

| cobra | down dog | yogi jumping jacks | yogi jumping jacks | yogi jumping jacks | yogi jumping jacks |
| *torso on floor* | | 1 | 2 | 3 | 4 |

| crescent | cat | tiger | cat | tiger | twisted child's pose |
| *leg lifted* | | *same arm/leg* | *forehead to knee* | *opposite arm/leg* | |

5-15 SETS

| four-limbed staff | down dog | plank | elevated thunderbolt | eight-angle pose | locust 1 |
| | | | *close eyes* | | |

WORK OUT

| hero | twisted hero | topsy-turvy | topsy-turvy | thunderbolt | tremulous |
| *close eyes* | | *opposite arm/leg* | *same arm/leg* | *hands bound* | *toes on floor* |

| down dog | mountain | crescent | lunge | high lunge | power pose |
| | | *triceps* | | | *hands bound* |

| crescent warrior | warrior 2 | eagle arms | warrior 1 | extended side angle | reverse warrior |
| | | | | *forearm on knee* | |

sequence 11 with Darren Rhodes

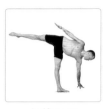
half moon
top arm in mountain

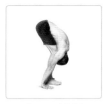
forward fold
knees bent

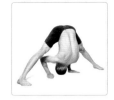
wide-leg forward fold

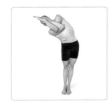
crescent
eagle arms

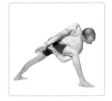
bound side angle

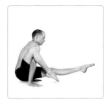
one-hand arm pose

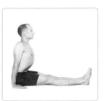
staff

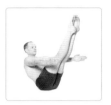
boat

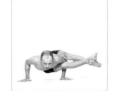
crooked sage
elbows bent

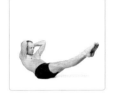
half boat

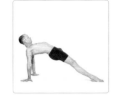
east stretch

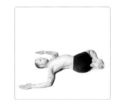
firmly rotated pose
knees bent

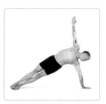
v sage
ankles stacked

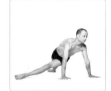
fallen sage
hips off floor

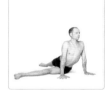
fallen sage
torso upright

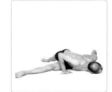
fallen sage

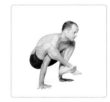
arm pressure pose

COOL DOWN

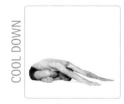
fire logs

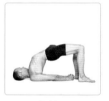
bridge

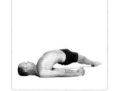
sideways
building bridge

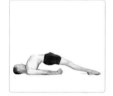
building bridge

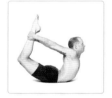
bow

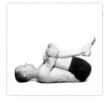
reclined child's pose

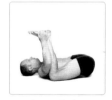
happy baby

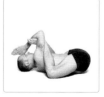
happy baby
palms together

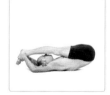
reclined west stretch

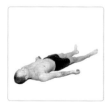
pose of repose

sequence 12 with Beth Daunis

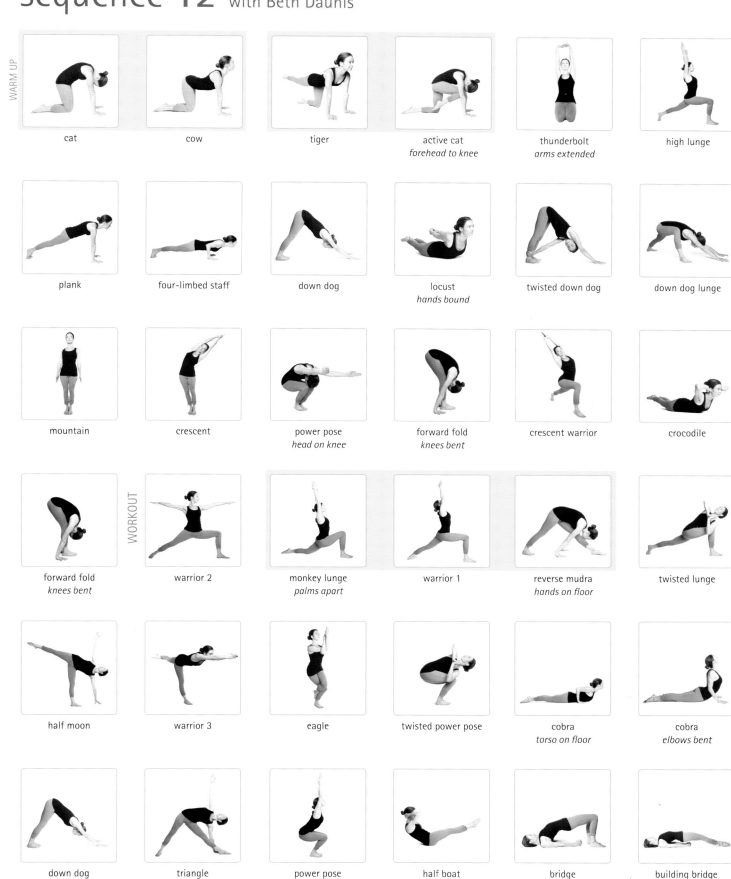

WARM UP

cat

cow

tiger

active cat
forehead to knee

thunderbolt
arms extended

high lunge

plank

four-limbed staff

down dog

locust
hands bound

twisted down dog

down dog lunge

mountain

crescent

power pose
head on knee

forward fold
knees bent

crescent warrior

crocodile

forward fold
knees bent

WORKOUT

warrior 2

monkey lunge
palms apart

warrior 1

reverse mudra
hands on floor

twisted lunge

half moon

warrior 3

eagle

twisted power pose

cobra
torso on floor

cobra
elbows bent

down dog

triangle

power pose

half boat

bridge

building bridge

sequence 12 with Beth Daunis

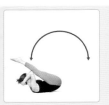

leg lifts
stage 1

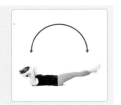

leg lifts
stage 2

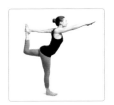

dancing yogi

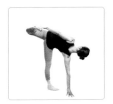

sugar cane

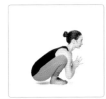

squat

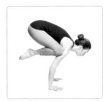

crane
shins parallel

reclined pigeon

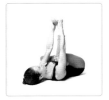

needle's eye

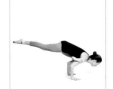

flying pigeon

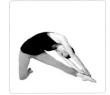

gate keeper

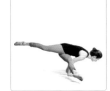

k sage 1

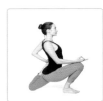

monkey lunge
quad stretch

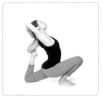

mermaid 2

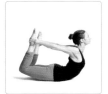

bow

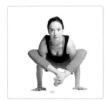

arm pressure pose

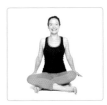

easy pose

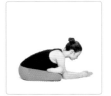

fire logs

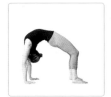

upward bow

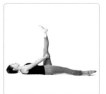

reclined big toe
prep

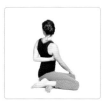

twisted sage 1

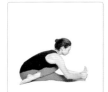

holy cow

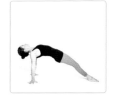

east stretch

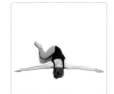

firmly rotated pose
knees bent

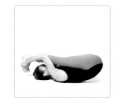

reclined west stretch

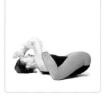

happy baby
palms together

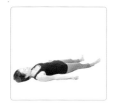

pose of repose

barefoot bootcamp Warm-up & Cool-down with Darren Rhodes

Warm-up

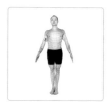
mountain

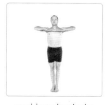
yogi jumping jacks
1

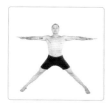
yogi jumping jacks
2

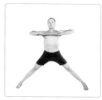
yogi jumping jacks
3

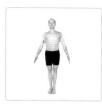
yogi jumping jacks
4

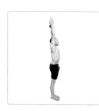
mountain
arms overhead

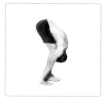
forward fold
knees bent

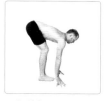
half forward fold
knees bent

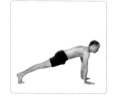
plank

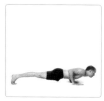
5 push-ups

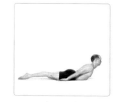
locust 1

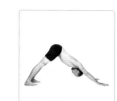
down dog

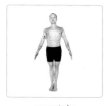
mountain
back of mat

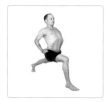
warrior 1
hands on hips

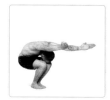
power pose
forehead to knee

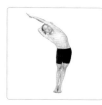
crescent
triceps

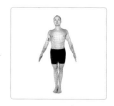
mountain
front of mat

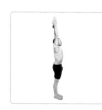
mountain
arms overhead

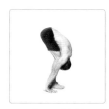
forward fold
knees bent

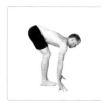
half forward fold
knees bent

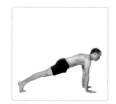
plank

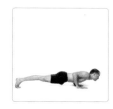
5 push-ups

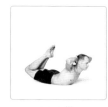
crocodile
knees bent

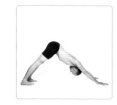
down dog

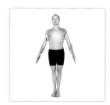
mountain
back of mat

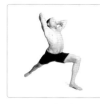
warrior 1
hands on head

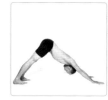
down dog

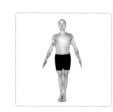
mountain
back of mat

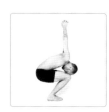
power pose
hands bound

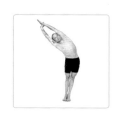
crescent
wrist

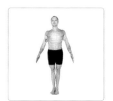
mountain
front of mat

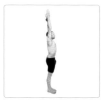
mountain
arms overhead

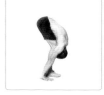
forward fold
knees bent

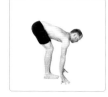
half forward fold
knees bent

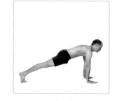
plank

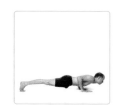
5 push-ups

Warm-up, cont.

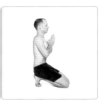

elevated thunderbolt

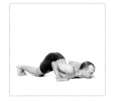

eight-angle pose

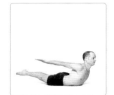

locust 2

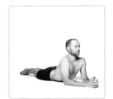

cobra
forearms on floor

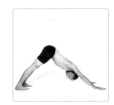

down dog

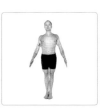

mountain
back of mat

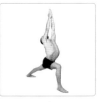

warrior 1

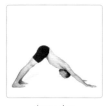

down dog

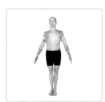

mountain
back of mat

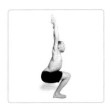

power pose

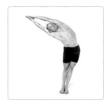

crescent

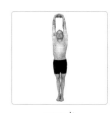

summit

crescent
leg lifted

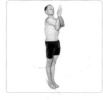

eagle arms

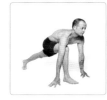

lunge

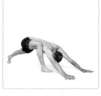

down dog lunge

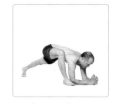

forearm lunge

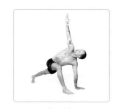

revolved lunge

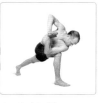

twisted lunge

Cool-down

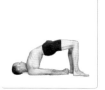

bridge

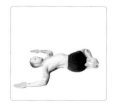

firmly rotated pose
knees bent

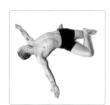

double diamond

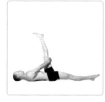

reclined big toe
prep

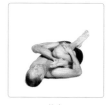

needle's eye

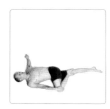

supine twist

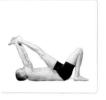

reclined bowing sage

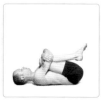

reclined child's pose

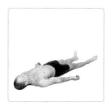

pose of repose

Standing & Supine

Begin this sequence with barefoot bootcamp Warm-Up (see separate sheet).
A cool down is incorporated into this sequence.

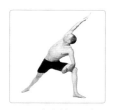
extended side angle
forearm on knee

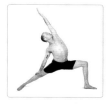
reverse warrior

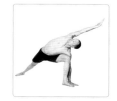
extended side angle

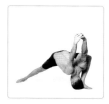
no-handed lunge

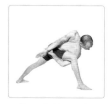
bound side angle

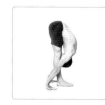
forward fold

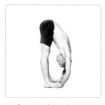
foot to hand pose

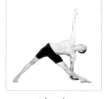
triangle

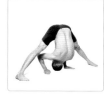
wide-leg forward fold

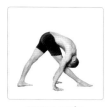
reverse mudra
hands on floor

revolved triangle

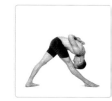
reverse mudra

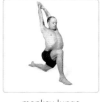
monkey lunge

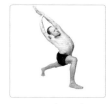
crescent warrior

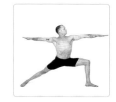
warrior 2

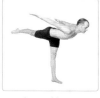
elevated locust

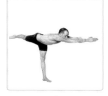
warrior 3

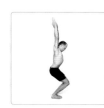
power pose
stage 2

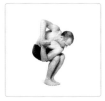
twisted power pose

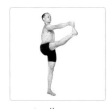
standing sage

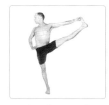
standing sage 2
look to side

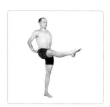
levitating sage

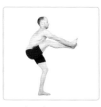
bowing sage
knees bent

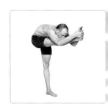
bowing sage

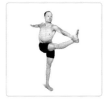
revolved sage

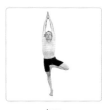
tree

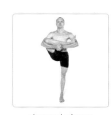
elevated pigeon

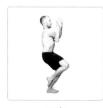
eagle

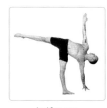
half moon

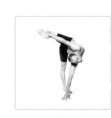
sugar cane

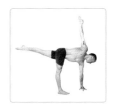
revolved half moon

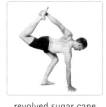
revolved sugar cane

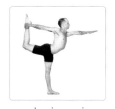
dancing yogi

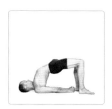
bridge

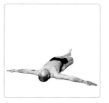
one-leg reclined hero

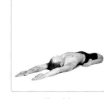
reclined hero

Standing & Supine, cont.

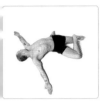
double diamond

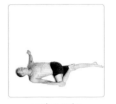
supine twist

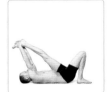
reclined bowing sage

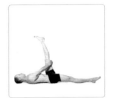
reclined big toe
prep

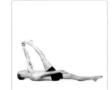
reclined big toe

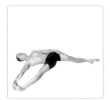
reclined big toe
leg to side

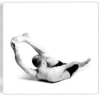
reclined big toe
forehead to knee

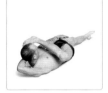
radical reclined big toe

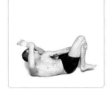
leg-behind-head
prep

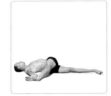
reclined revolved sage

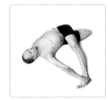
Tibetan weaponry 3

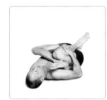
needle's eye

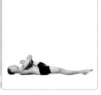
reclined pigeon

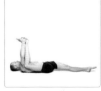
reclined lunge

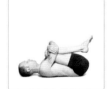
reclined child's pose

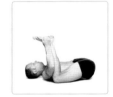
happy baby

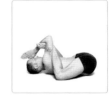
happy baby
palms together

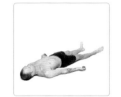
pose of repose

Arm Balances

Begin this sequence with barefoot bootcamp Warm-Up (see separate sheet).
End with barefoot bootcamp Cool Down.

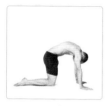
cat

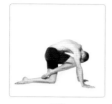
cat
forehead to knee

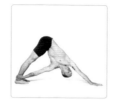
twisted down dog

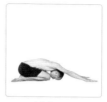
child's pose

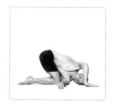
twisted child's pose

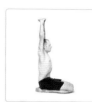
thunderbolt
arms extended

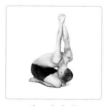
thunderbolt
hands bound

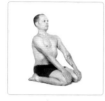
hero

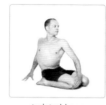
twisted hero

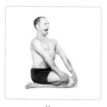
lion

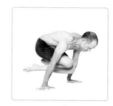
tremulous

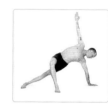
v sage
foot on floor

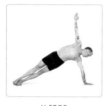
v sage
ankles stacked

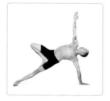
tree sage 1

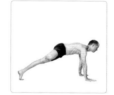
plank
leg in tree

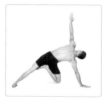
tree sage 2

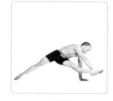
v sage
hold bottom foot

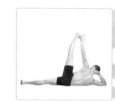
endless pose

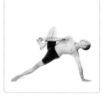
v sage
knee bent

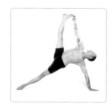
v sage

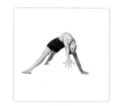
wild thing

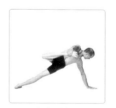
baby bird

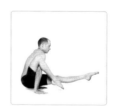
one-hand arm pose

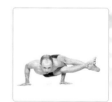
crooked sage
arms bent

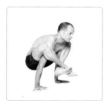
arm pressure pose

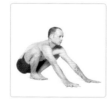
squat

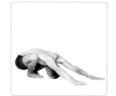
garland 1

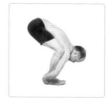
garland 2
stage 1

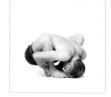
garland 2

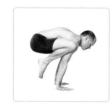
crane
thighs parallel

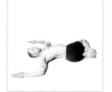
firmly rotated pose
knees bent

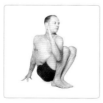
noose
elbow bent

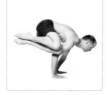
turned crane

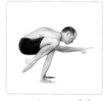
one-leg crane (b.)

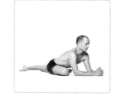
pigeon

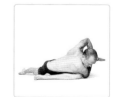
twisted pigeon 1

Arm Balances, cont.

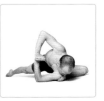
twisted pigeon 2

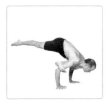
flying pigeon

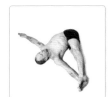
firmly rotated pose

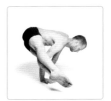
two-leg k sage

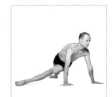
fallen sage
hips off floor

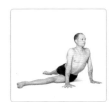
fallen sage
torso upright

fallen sage

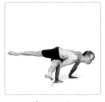
k sage 1

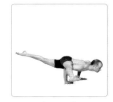
k sage 2

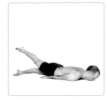
inverted locust
leg lifted

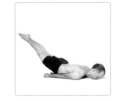
inverted locust

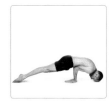
peacock
head on floor

peacock
head off floor

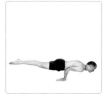
peacock

End with barefoot bootcamp Cool-down.

Forward Folds

Begin this sequence with barefoot bootcamp Warm-Up (see separate sheet).
End with barefoot bootcamp Cool Down.

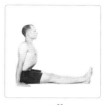
staff

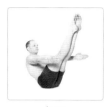
boat

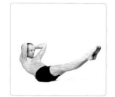
half boat

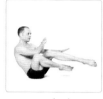
cosmic abs

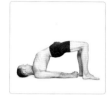
bridge

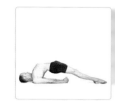
building bridge

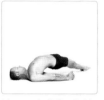
sideways building bridge

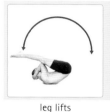
leg lifts
stage 1

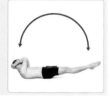
leg lifts
stage 2

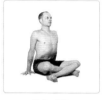
easy pose
torso upright

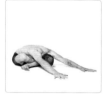
easy pose

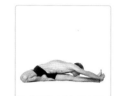
head knee pose

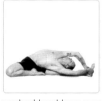
revolved head knee pose

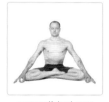
accomplished pose

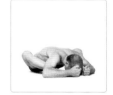
star

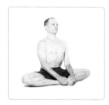
bound angle
torso upright

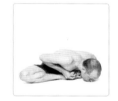
bound angle

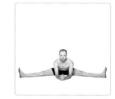
seated angle
forearms on floor

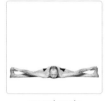
seated angle

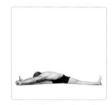
lateral seated angle

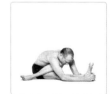
holy cow pose

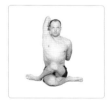
cow face 1
torso upright

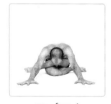
cow face 1
forward fold

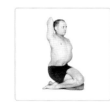
cow face 2

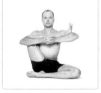
seated pigeon

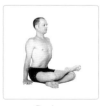
fire logs
torso upright

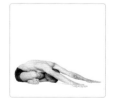
fire logs

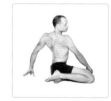
twisted sage
stage 1

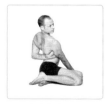
twisted sage

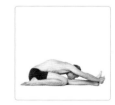
triad

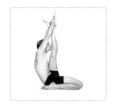
heron

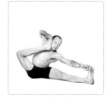
archer 1

archer 2

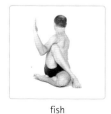
fish
elbow bent

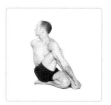
fish

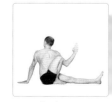
revolved m sage 1
elbow bent

Forward Folds, cont.

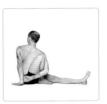
revolved m sage 1
clasp wrist

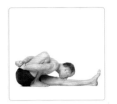
m sage 1

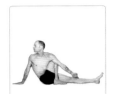
m sage 3
hand to shin

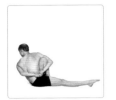
m sage 3

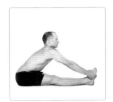
west stretch
spine extended

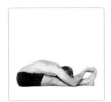
west stretch

both big toes pose

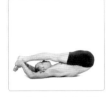
reclined west stretch

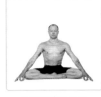
meditation pose

End with barefoot bootcamp Cool-down.

barefoot bootcamp with Darren Rhodes

Backbends

Begin this sequence with barefoot bootcamp Warm-Up (see separate sheet).
End with barefoot bootcamp Cool-down.

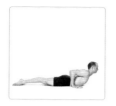
cobra
torso on floor

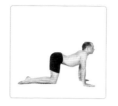
cow

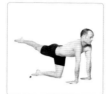
southpaw tiger

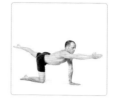
tiger
opposite arm/leg

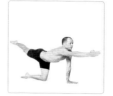
tiger
same arm/leg

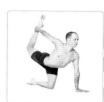
elevated bow
same arm/leg

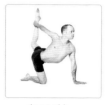
elevated bow
opposite arm/leg

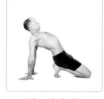
thunderbolt
quad stretch

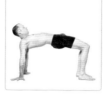
reverse table

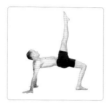
reverse table
leg lifted

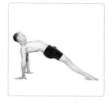
east stretch

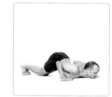
eight-angle pose

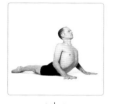
cobra
elbows bent

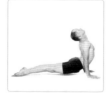
up dog

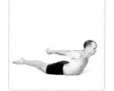
locust
hands bound

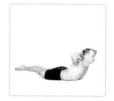
crocodile

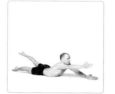
topsy-turvy
opposite arm/leg

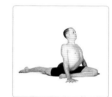
pigeon
torso upright

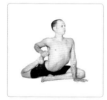
pigeon quad stretch

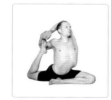
mermaid 1

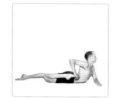
half frog

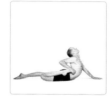
elevated half frog

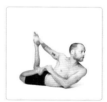
gherandasana 1
prep

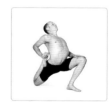
monkey lunge
quad stretch

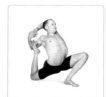
mermaid 2

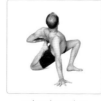
twisted monkey

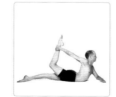
one-leg bow

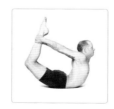
bow

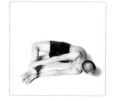
sideways bow

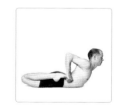
frog

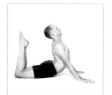
king pigeon
shins vertical

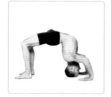
upward bow
head on floor

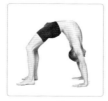
upward bow

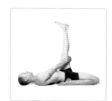
Tibetan weaponry 1

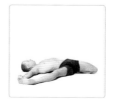
Tibetan weaponry 2

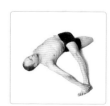
Tibetan weaponry 3

Backbends, cont.

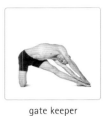
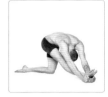
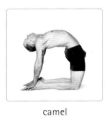
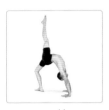
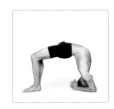

gate keeper   kneeling sage   camel   upward bow   inverted staff
                                                           leg lifted

End with barefoot bootcamp Cool-down.

yogahour syllabus

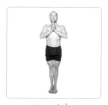
mountain
palms together

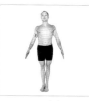
mountain

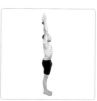
mountain
arms overhead

summit

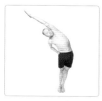
crescent
hand on hip

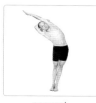
crescent
triceps

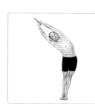
crescent
wrist

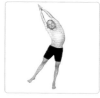
crescent
leg lifted

crescent

crescent
eagle arms

forward fold
knees bent

forward fold

half forward fold
knees bent

half forward fold

foot to hand pose
knees bent

foot to hand pose

hands to big toe
knees bent

hands to big toe

hands to big toe
extended spine

extended side angle
forearm on knee

extended side angle
hand on block

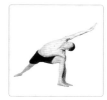
extended side angle

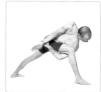
bound side angle

lunge

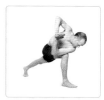
twisted lunge

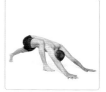
down dog lunge

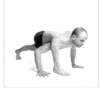
crouching warrior

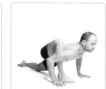
crouching monkey

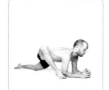
forearm lunge
knee on floor

forearm lunge

revolved lunge
knee on floor

revolved lunge

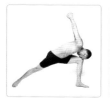
no-handed lunge
head to knee

no-handed lunge

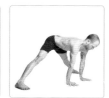
wide-leg forward fold
hands under shoulders

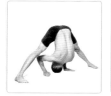
wide-leg forward fold

triangle
hand on block

triangle
look down

triangle

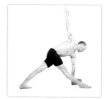
revolved triangle
hand on block

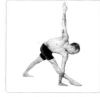
revolved triangle
look down

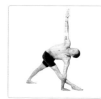
revolved triangle

yogahour syllabus

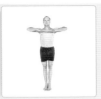
yogi jumping jacks
1

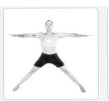
yogi jumping jacks
2

yogi jumping jacks
3

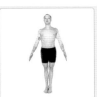
yogi jumping jacks
4

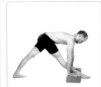
reverse mudra
hands on blocks

reverse mudra
hands on floor

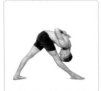
reverse mudra

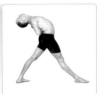
reverse mudra
backbend

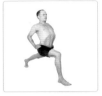
warrior 1
hands on hips

high lunge

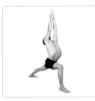
warrior 1

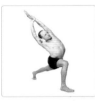
crescent warrior

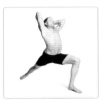
warrior 1
hands on head

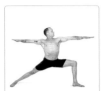
warrior 2

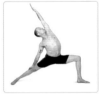
reverse warrior

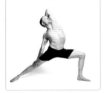
reverse warrior
hand to head

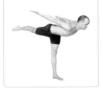
elevated locust

elevated locust
hands bound

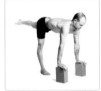
warrior 3
hands on blocks

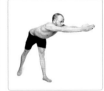
warrior 3
leg lifts

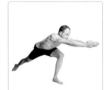
warrior 3
back foot on floor

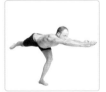
warrior 3
knee bent

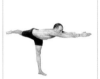
warrior 3

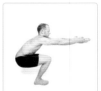
power pose
stage 1

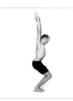
power pose
stage 2

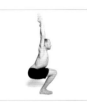
power pose

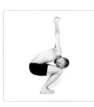
power pose
hands bound

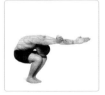
power pose
head to knee

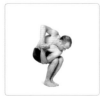
twisted power pose

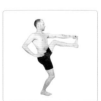
standing sage
knees bent

standing sage

standing sage 2
top knee bent

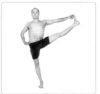
standing sage 2

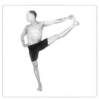
standing sage 2
look to side

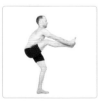
bowing sage
knees bent

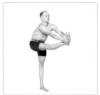
bowing sage
stage 1

bowing sage

revolved sage
knees bent

revolved sage

levitating sage

tree
*palms together, hands
to heart*

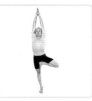
tree

yogahour syllabus

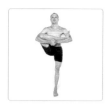
elevated pigeon

mountain
eagle arms

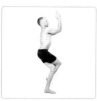
eagle
forearms together

eagle

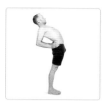
standing camel

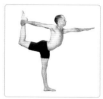
dancing yogi

dancing yogi
hands on ankle

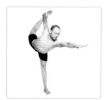
dancing warrior 3

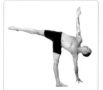
half moon

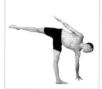
half moon
top arm in mountain

sugar cane

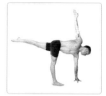
revolved half moon

revolved sugar cane
heel to hip

revolved sugar cane

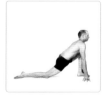
monkey lunge
hands on floor

monkey lunge
palms apart

monkey lunge

monkey lunge
hands on head

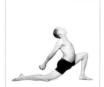
monkey lunge
hands bound

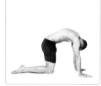
cat

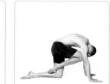
cat
forehead to knee

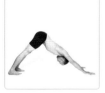
down dog

down dog
leg lifted

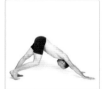
down dog jog

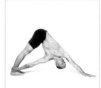
twisted down dog

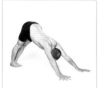
down dog
ankles together

child's pose

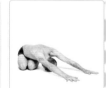
sideways child's pose

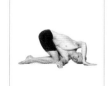
twisted child's pose

squat

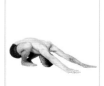
garland 1

garland 2
stage 1

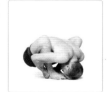
garland 2

formidable forearm
pose

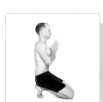
elevated thunderbolt

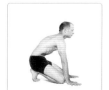
thunderbolt
toe crusher

thunderbolt
arms extended

thunderbolt
hands bound

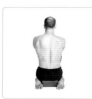
hero
hips on block

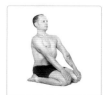
hero

twisted hero

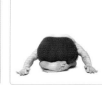
fallen hero

yogahour syllabus

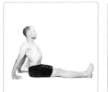
staff
hands behind hips

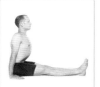
staff

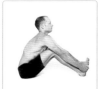
west stretch
knees bent

west stretch
spine extended

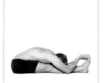
west stretch

both big toes pose

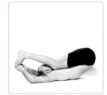
reclined west stretch
knees bent

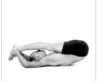
reclined west stretch

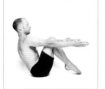
boat
stage 1

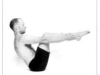
boat
stage 2

boat

half boat
stage 1

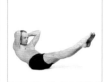
half boat

cosmic abs

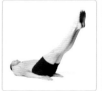
leg lifts
hands under hips

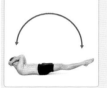
leg lifts
stage 1

leg lifts
stage 2

leg lifts, stage 1
twist variation

leg lifts, stage 2
twist variation

easy pose
torso upright

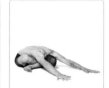
easy pose

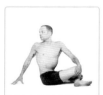
twisted easy pose

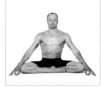
meditation pose

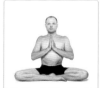
OM pose

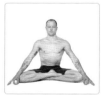
accomplished pose

bound angle
torso upright

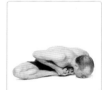
bound angle

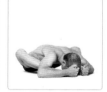
star

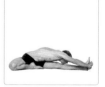
head knee pose

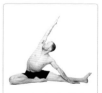
revolved head knee
stage 1

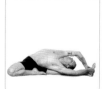
revolved head knee

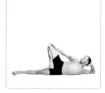
endless pose
foot in tree

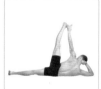
endless pose

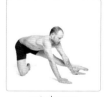
gate keeper
stage 1

gate keeper
stage 2

gate keeper

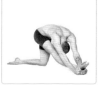
kneeling sage

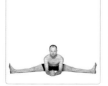
seated angle
forearms on floor

seated angle

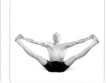
elevated seated angle

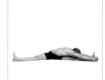
lateral seated angle

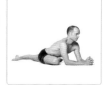
pigeon

yogahour syllabus

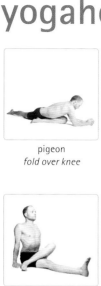
pigeon
fold over knee

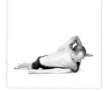
twisted pigeon 1

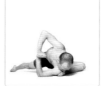
twisted pigeon 2

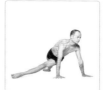
fallen sage
hips off floor

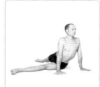
fallen sage
torso upright

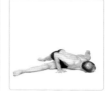
fallen sage

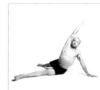
fallen sage
crescent stretch

holy cow
torso upright

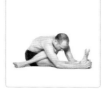
holy cow pose

cow face 1
fold forward

cow face 1
torso upright

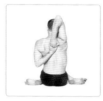
cow face 1
torso upright

cow face 2

seated pigeon
leg straight

seated pigeon

fire logs
torso upright

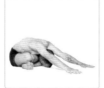
fire logs

twisted sage
stage 1

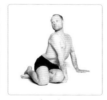
twisted sage
stage 2

twisted sage

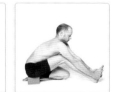
triad
hips on block

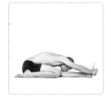
triad

heron
hips on block

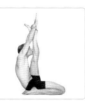
heron

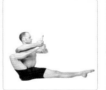
archer 1
stage 1

archer 1

archer 2
hand on floor

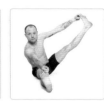
archer 2
stage 1

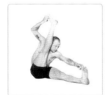
archer 2

fish
elbow bent

fish

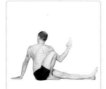
revolved m sage 1
elbow bent

revolved m sage 1
clasp wrist

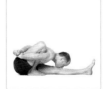
m sage 1

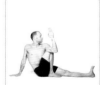
m sage 3
elbow bent

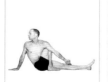
m sage 3
hand to shin

m sage 3

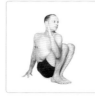
noose
elbow bent

one-leg noose

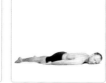
prone
pose of repose

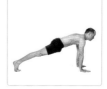
plank

plank
leg lifted

yogahour syllabus

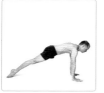
plank
feet pointed

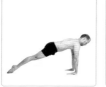
southpaw plank
feet pointed

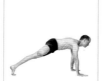
plank
leg in tree

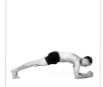
forearm plank

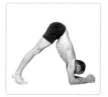
dolphin

four-limbed staff

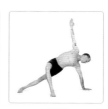
v sage
foot on floor

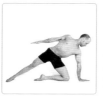
v sage
knee on floor

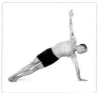
v sage
ankles stacked

tree sage 1

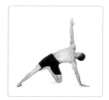
tree sage 2

v sage
knee bent

v sage

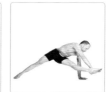
v sage
hold bottom foot

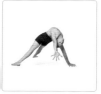
wild thing

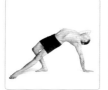
wild thing
hand on head

baby bird
knee on floor

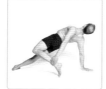
baby bird
foot on floor

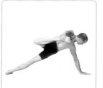
baby bird

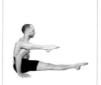
one-hand arm pose
stage 1

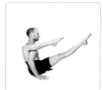
one-hand arm pose
stage 2

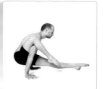
one-hand arm pose
stage 3

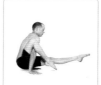
one-hand arm pose

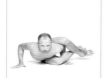
crooked sage
hips on floor

crooked sage
feet on floor

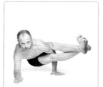
crooked sage
forearm on floor

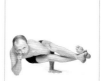
crooked sage
hand to chin

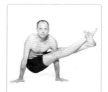
crooked sage
arms straight

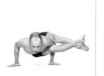
crooked sage
arms bent

lion

tremulous
toes on floor

tremulous

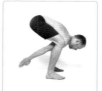
arm pressure pose
stage 1

arm pressure pose
stage 2

arm pressure pose
stage 3

arm pressure pose

arm pressure pose
head on floor

crane
elbows bent

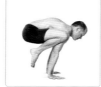
crane
thighs parallel

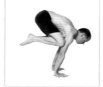
crane
shins parallel

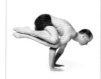
turned crane

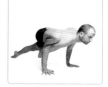
one-leg crane (a.)
foot on floor

yogahour syllabus

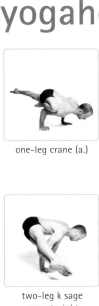
one-leg crane (a.)

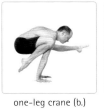
one-leg crane (b.)

nesting pigeon

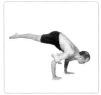
flying pigeon

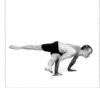
k sage 1

wild card pose

k sage 2

two-leg k sage
arm straight

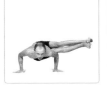
two-leg k sage

peacock
head on floor

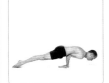
peacock
head off floor

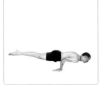
peacock

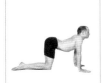
cow

tiger

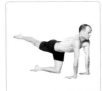
southpaw tiger

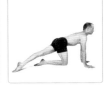
tiger
leg lifts

tiger
opposite arm/leg

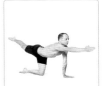
tiger
same arm/leg

elevated bow
opposite arm/leg

elevated bow
same arm/leg

thunderbolt
quad stretch

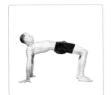
reverse table

reverse table
knee bent

reverse table
shin parallel

reverse table
leg vertical

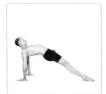
east stretch

eight-angle pose

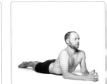
cobra
forearms on floor

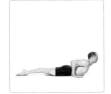
cobra
torso on floor

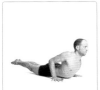
cobra
legs off floor

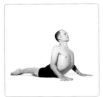
cobra
elbows bent

up dog

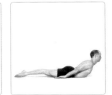
locust 1

locust 1
knees bent

locust 2

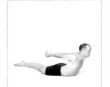
locust
hands bound

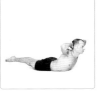
crocodile

crocodile
knees bent

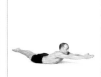
superhero

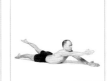
topsy-turvy
opposite arm/leg

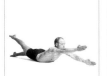
topsy-turvy
same arm/leg

inverted locust
knees bent

yogahour syllabus

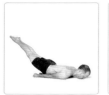 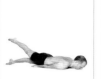 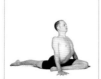 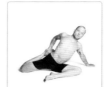 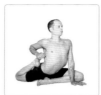 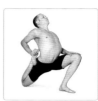

| inverted locust | inverted locust *one leg lifted* | pigeon *torso upright* | pigeon quad stretch *hip on floor* | pigeon *quad stretch* | mermaid 1 | monkey lunge *quad stretch* |

 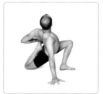 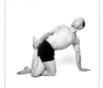 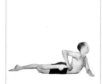 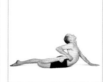 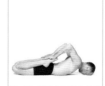 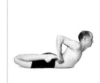

| mermaid 2 | twisted monkey | funky monkey | half frog | elevated half frog | frog *head on floor* | frog |

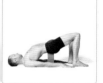 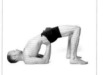 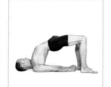 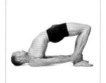

| bridge *block under hips* | bridge *hands on hips* | sideways bridge *hand on hip* | bridge | bridge *quad stretch* | bridge *hold ankles* | sideways bridge |

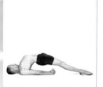 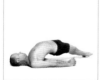 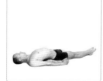 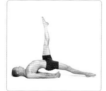 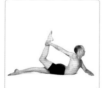

| building bridge | sideways building bridge | fallen bridge | building bridge *leg lifted* | one-leg bow | gherandasana 1 *prep* | bow |

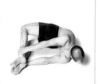 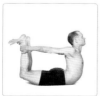 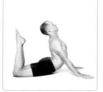   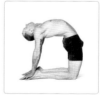 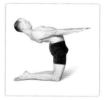

| sideways bow | bow *feet flexed* | king pigeon *shins vertical* | camel *hands on hips* | camel *look straight ahead* | camel | camel reps |

   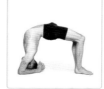 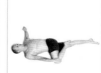 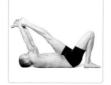 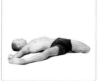

| upward bow *head on floor* | upward bow | upward bow *leg lifted* | inverted staff | supine twist | reclined bowing sage | Tibetan weaponry 2 |

yogahour syllabus

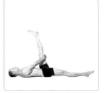
reclined big toe
prep

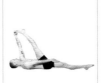
reclined big toe

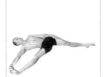
reclined big toe
leg to side

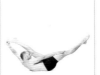
reclined big toe
*forehead to knee,
foot off floor*

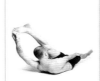
reclined big toe
forehead to knee

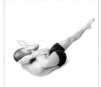
radical reclined big toe
prep

radical reclined big toe
clasp wrist

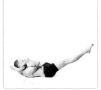
radical reclined big toe
hands bound

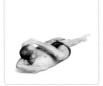
radical reclined big toe

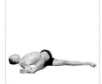
reclined revolved sage

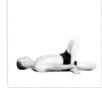
Tibetan weaponry 3
prep

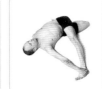
Tibetan weaponry 3

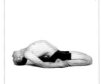
couch pose
prep

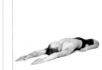
reclined hero

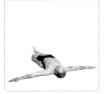
one-leg
reclined hero

Tibetan weaponry 1

reclined eagle

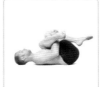
reclined cow face

needle's eye

needle's eye
shin vertical

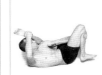
leg-behind-head
prep

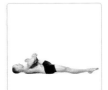
reclined pigeon

firmly rotated pose
knees bent

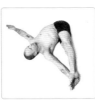
firmly rotated pose

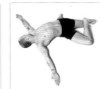
double diamond

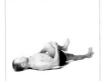
one leg reclined
child's pose

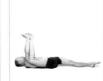
reclined lunge

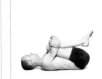
reclined child's pose

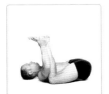
happy baby

happy baby
palms together

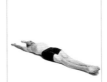
reclined mountain
arms overhead

pose of repose

NOTES:

NOTES: